Mahdi Manoochehri
Zahra Azadifard
Asrin Hemmatboland

The Effect of Lifestyle on Cancer

Mahdi Manoochehri
Zahra Azadifard
Asrin Hemmatboland

The Effect of Lifestyle on Cancer

(Breast Cancer Study)

Noor Publishing

Imprint

Any brand names and product names mentioned in this book are subject to trademark, brand or patent protection and are trademarks or registered trademarks of their respective holders. The use of brand names, product names, common names, trade names, product descriptions etc. even without a particular marking in this work is in no way to be construed to mean that such names may be regarded as unrestricted in respect of trademark and brand protection legislation and could thus be used by anyone.

Cover image: www.ingimage.com

Publisher:
Noor Publishing
is a trademark of
Dodo Books Indian Ocean Ltd., member of the OmniScriptum S.R.L Publishing group
str. A.Russo 15, of. 61, Chisinau-2068, Republic of Moldova Europe
Printed at: see last page
ISBN: 978-620-3-86042-9

The Effect of Lifestyle on Cancer (Breast Cancer Study)

By

Mahdi Manoochehri

Master student of Medical-Surgical Nursing, Iran University of Medical Sciences, Iran

Zahra Azadifard

Master Student of Community Health, Lorestan University of Medical Sciences, Iran

Asrin Hemmatboland

Nursing Expert, Islamic Azad University, Maragheh Branch, Maragheh, Iran

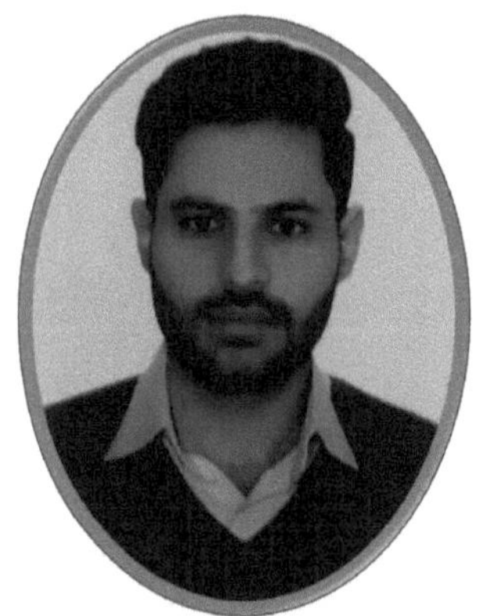

Mahdi Manoochehri

Master student of Medical-Surgical Nursing, Iran University of Medical Sciences, Iran

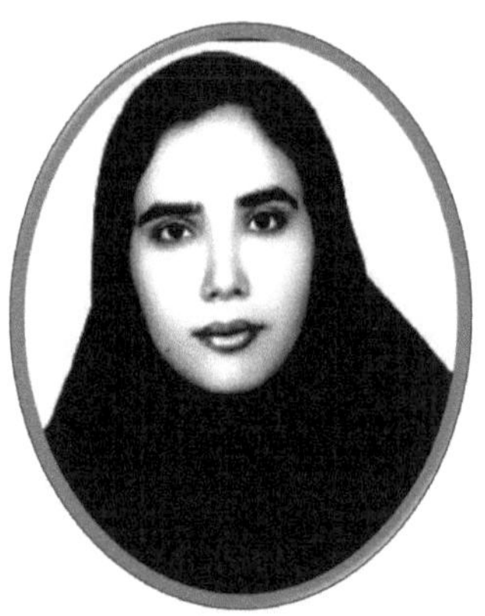

Zahra Azadifard

Master Student of Community Health, Lorestan University of Medical Sciences, Iran

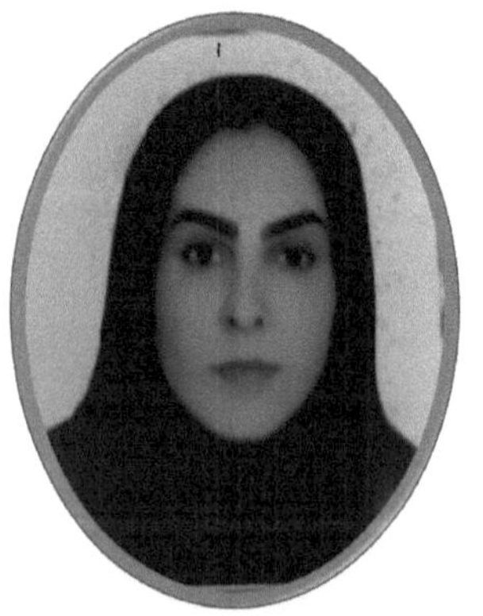

Asrin Hemmatboland

Nursing Expert, Islamic Azad University, Maragheh Branch, Maragheh, Iran

This Book is dedicated to

My Family's

Content

Chapter I

Introduction

Cancer

Cancer means the abnormal growth, proliferation and sometimes proliferation of cells in the body. All cancers have an uncontrolled growth pattern and a tendency to detach from the original source and metastasize.

General overview

The human body is made up of millions upon millions of cells that work together to build tissues such as muscles, bones and skin. Most of the body's natural cells grow and reproduce in response to stimuli from inside and outside the body, and eventually die. If this process takes place in a balanced and correct way, the body will remain healthy and maintain its normal function. But problems start when a normal cell mutates or changes into a cancer cell.

How cancer develops

A normal cell may turn into a cancer cell for no apparent reason, but in most cases, it is the result of repeated exposure to carcinogens such as alcohol and tobacco. The appearance and function of cancer cells are different from normal cells. A mutation or change in the DNA or genetic material of a cell occurs. DNA is responsible for controlling the appearance and function of cells. When a cell's DNA changes, that cell differentiates from the healthy cells next to it and no longer does the body's normal cells. This altered cell separates from its neighboring cells and does not know when it should stop growing and die. In other words, the altered cell does not follow the internal commands and signals that other cells are in control of and acts arbitrarily instead of coordinating with other cells.

Malignant cancer

When a mutant cell divides, it becomes two new mutant cells, and the process continues in the same way until the same insidious cell turns into a mass of cells called a tumor. Sometimes these tumors are benign and do not grow. But if the tumor cells grow and divide and destroy the normal cells around them and reach other parts of the body, the tumor is considered malignant. The greatest risk of malignant tumors is their ability to invade healthy tissues and spread throughout the body, and this is cancer metastasis. As the tumors grow and enlarge, they prevent nutrients and oxygen from reaching healthy cells, and as healthy cancer progresses, healthy cells die and the patient's function and health are lost. If this process is not stopped, cancer can lead to death.

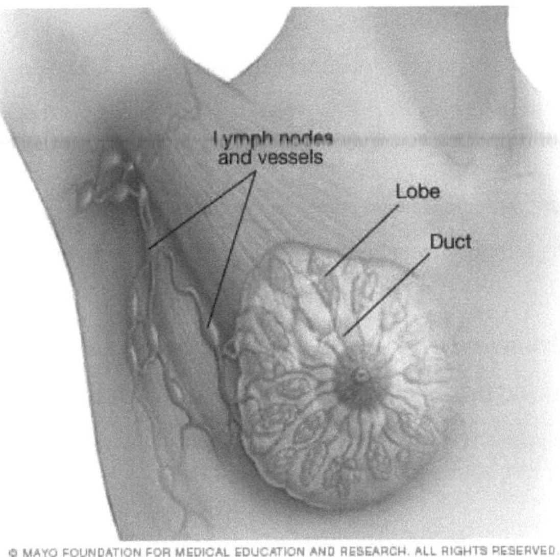

Figure 1. Breast cancer - Symptoms and causes

Cancer warning signs

- ✓ Abnormal bleeding anywhere on the body.
- ✓ The appearance of any solid cell mass under the skin, for example in the breast or elsewhere.
- ✓ The appearance of a wound that does not heal easily (odor around the tongue, mouth and lips).
- ✓ Persistent indigestion.
- ✓ Changes in the condition of moles or warts such as discoloration, enlargement, itching, pain, or bleeding that last for a long time.
- ✓ Disorders of bowel or bladder function that do not improve with normal treatment.

✓ Cough, hoarseness or difficulty swallowing for a long time.

✓ If any of these symptoms persist for more than two weeks, the patient should be examined professionally. Of course, in most cases, these symptoms do not indicate the presence of cancer.

Types of cancers

Most cancers fall into three main categories:

Carcinoma: Includes cancers that originate from cells that make up the skin (such as skin cancer) or cover the lining of the organs (such as lung cancer) or that make up the glands (such as breast cancer).

Sarcoma: These are cancers that originate in connective tissue such as cartilage, bone, and muscle. This is why bone cancer or muscle cancer anywhere in the body is called sarcoma.

Leukemias and lymphomas: These include cancers that originate in the cells that make up the blood and the immune cells. Skin cancer is the most common cancer in Western countries, followed by breast, lung, prostate, colon, bladder and uterine cancers.

Ways of prevention

Primary cancer prevention is done by avoiding the causative agent or consuming substances that prevent the onset of the malignant process, and includes measures to reduce lifestyle risks (avoiding tobacco, eating low-fat, high-fiber foods, and using sunscreen). And the use of chemical preventative agents. Chemical inhibitors are drugs or micronutrients (minerals or vitamins). The following factors are also effective in preventing cancer.

✓ Do not use alcohol and tobacco.

✓ Eat foods that are cooked.

✓ Do not use foods that show signs of burns.

✓ Use vegetables and fruits.

✓ Use less red meat.

✓ Full observance of health affairs.

Treatment

Most cancers today have no definitive cure, but surgery, radiation therapy, chemotherapy, hormone therapy, and bone marrow transplantation are used to prevent them from growing and progressing. However, new findings in tumor cell biology are being used in combination therapies in a coordinated program.

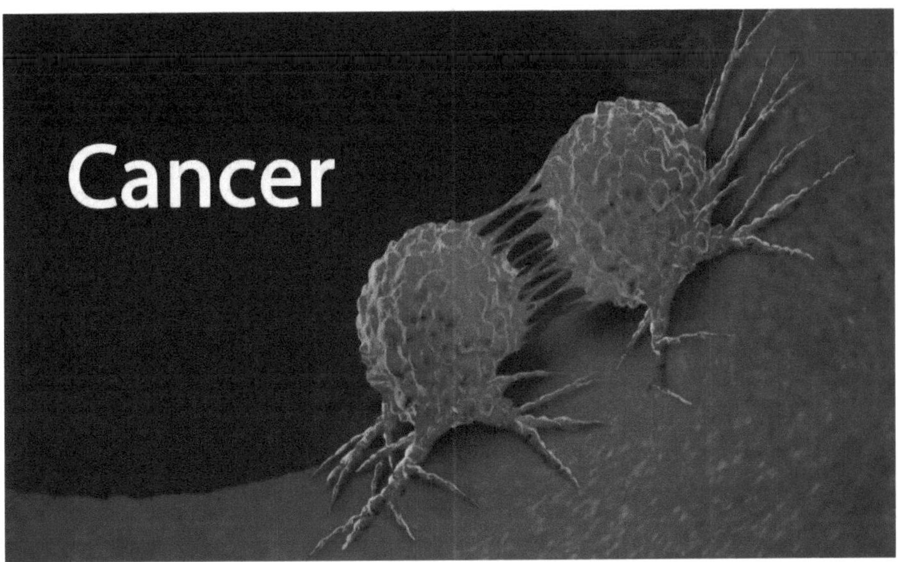

Figure 2. Anti-nausea drug may help cancer patients survive longer

Facts About Lung Cancer

What is lung cancer?

Lung cancer is the most common cause of cancer death in both men and women. It seems. It is less common in some races, such as white men and African-American men. There are generally two types of lung cancer.

What are the causes of lung cancer?

The main cause of lung cancer is smoking. Cigarette smoke contains more than 4,000 types of chemicals, most of which are carcinogenic. Any other device such as a pipe or hookah has similar conditions to cigarettes. The longer you smoke and the more you smoke per day, the higher your chances of getting cancer. But if you stop smoking annually, your chances of getting cancer will be significantly reduced. After 10 years of quitting, the chances of getting 1.3 to half of those who still smoke will increase. In addition, quitting smoking will significantly reduce other smoking-related diseases such as heart disease, stroke, emphysema and chronic bronchitis. In addition, many of the chemicals in cigarettes can be dangerous to those who are indirectly exposed to them, leading to lung cancer. Radon gas appears to be the second leading cause of lung cancer in the United States. This gas can easily spread through the walls of houses and through pipes and municipal sewage, and since one cannot see or smell it, the only way to evaluate a person with this gas is to measure it. Exposure to radon along with smoking significantly increases the chances of developing lung cancer. Another cause of lung cancer is exposure to chemicals in the workplace. Asbestosis is one of the known substances in this group. But in addition to other substances such as uranium, arsenic and some petroleum products should be mentioned. The chances of developing lung cancer are multiplied when work-related exposure is associated with smoking. Lung cancer takes a long time to grow. But changes in the lungs begin almost immediately after exposure to carcinogens. Immediately after the start of contact, a number of special cells are placed inside the lining of the airways. These cells are abnormal and if more contact continues, more cells will form and cause cancer.

How is lung cancer diagnosed?

In the early stages of this cancer, it does not cause any symptoms. Cancer is usually advanced when symptoms appear. Symptoms of lung cancer include chronic cough, hoarseness, sputum with blood, weight loss and loss of appetite, shortness of breath, fever without any obvious symptoms, wheezing, recurrence of diseases such as bronchitis or pneumonia, and chest pain. These symptoms may also be present in other lung diseases. Therefore, if you have these symptoms, you should see a doctor to determine the cause. When a person comes for an examination, the doctor will ask them different questions about the person's medical history as well as contact with carcinogens, in addition to examining the patient. If the patient has a sputum cough, the sputum should be checked for cancer. In addition, a chest x-ray or CT scan may be requested to detect any abnormalities in the lungs. In addition, a device called a bronchoscope may be used to look directly at the airways and lungs and to sample or biopsy the tumor. All of these are some of the ways in which lung cancer can be diagnosed.

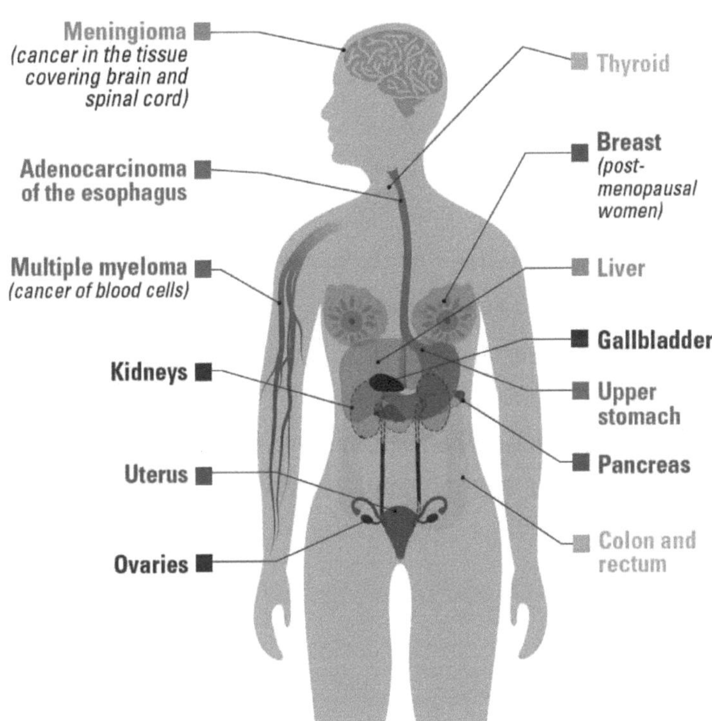

Figure 3. Obesity and Cancer

A special type of CT scan may be used to detect very small cancers that have a better chance of being cured. The set of studies performed on diagnostic methods shows its effectiveness in early detection of cancers, even in small sizes. If cancer is diagnosed, other tests should be done to see if the cancer has spread to other parts of the body. This information helps the doctor choose the best treatment. These tests include CT scans, MRIs, and bone scans.

How is lung cancer treated?

The type of treatment chosen for lung cancer varies depending on the type of cancer, the size of the tumor, its location and extent, and the general condition of the patient. There are several treatments that can be used alone or in combination, including the following.

Surgery: This method is used in the early stages of cancer. The type of surgery depends on the location of the tumor. Some cancers cannot be surgically removed because of their size and location.

Radiation therapy: These methods use high-energy X-rays to kill cancer cells. This method can be used in combination with chemotherapy or surgery. Using this method, airway pain and obstruction can be relieved.

Chemotherapy: In this method, special drugs are used to fight cancer. These drugs can be injected through a vein, But its oral forms are also available. This method can be used in conjunction with surgery. In addition, it can be used in advanced stages of cancer to relieve symptoms. This method can also be used in all stages of small cell cancer.

How can lung cancer be prevented?

✓ If you are a smoker, quit.

✓ If you are not a smoker, stay in the workplace or public areas free of smoke or any contaminants.

✓ Avoid cigarette smoke in the house.

✓ If you are exposed to dust and fumes in the workplace, ask how you protect yourself.

✓ Never smoke because you will be much more likely to get it if you work in polluted environments.

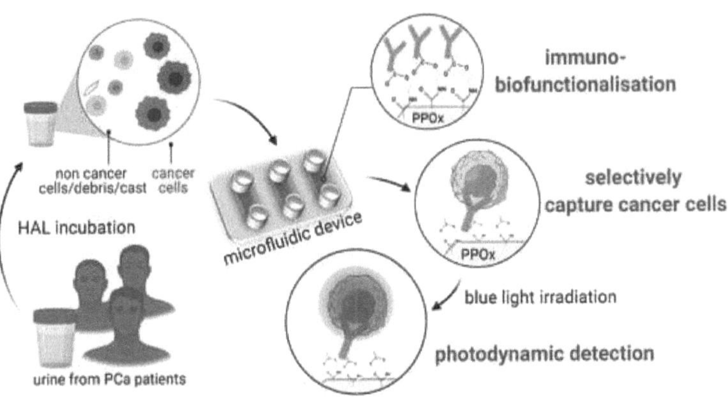

Figure 4. Cancers

Colon cancer

What is colon cancer?

In this disease, cancer cells begin to multiply inside the intestinal tissue. Although this cancer is one of the most common human cancers, but due to improved screening and diagnostic methods, the number of new cases of this disease and the resulting deaths have decreased significantly. It can occur at any age, but is more common in people over the age of 50. When diagnosed in the early stages, this cancer is treatable but its diagnosis in these stages has no symptoms. The large intestine is part of the digestive system, including the esophagus, stomach, large and small intestines. The small intestine starts at the end of the stomach and ends in the large intestine, and then the large intestine continues from there to the anus. The large intestine consists of two parts. The first part is called the colon. Which is about 180 cm long. The second part is the rectum, which is 15 to 25 cm long.

Risk factors

The following factors may increase a person's chances of developing colon cancer.

- ✓ **Age:** Most people with this disease are over 50 years old, but it can occur at any age.
- ✓ **Diet:** There is a direct relationship between this disease and a diet high in fat, high in energy and low in fiber.
- ✓ **Polyps:** This disease is defined as the growth of benign masses in the intestinal wall, which is usually common after the age of 50 years. This structure appears to increase the chances of developing colon cancer.
- ✓ **Personal history:** People who have had colon cancer before, or women who have had ovarian, uterine, or breast cancer, are more likely to develop the disease. At present, in some cases of this cancer, the responsible genes have been identified. Therefore, before cancer, such people are examined for gene expression.
- ✓ **Ulcerative colitis:** In this disease, the lining of the colon is inflamed. People with this disease are more likely to get it.

Signs and symptoms

The symptoms of this disease may be similar to other symptoms such as infections, hemorrhoids and inflammatory bowel disease. Therefore, it is necessary to see a doctor for a better evaluation. Since in the early stages of the disease can be successfully treated. See your doctor if you notice any of the following symptoms.

- ✓ Any change in bowel defecation habits such as diarrhea, constipation or decreased stool diameter that lasts more than a day.
- ✓ Bleeding from the rectum or the presence of blood in the stool.

✓ Colic pains in the stomach.

✓ Vomiting.

✓ Weakness and fatigue.

✓ Jaundice and jaundice of the skin or sclera (whites of the eyes).

In some cases, the person may have cancer but no symptoms. Therefore, screening in high-risk individuals such as those over 50 is essential.

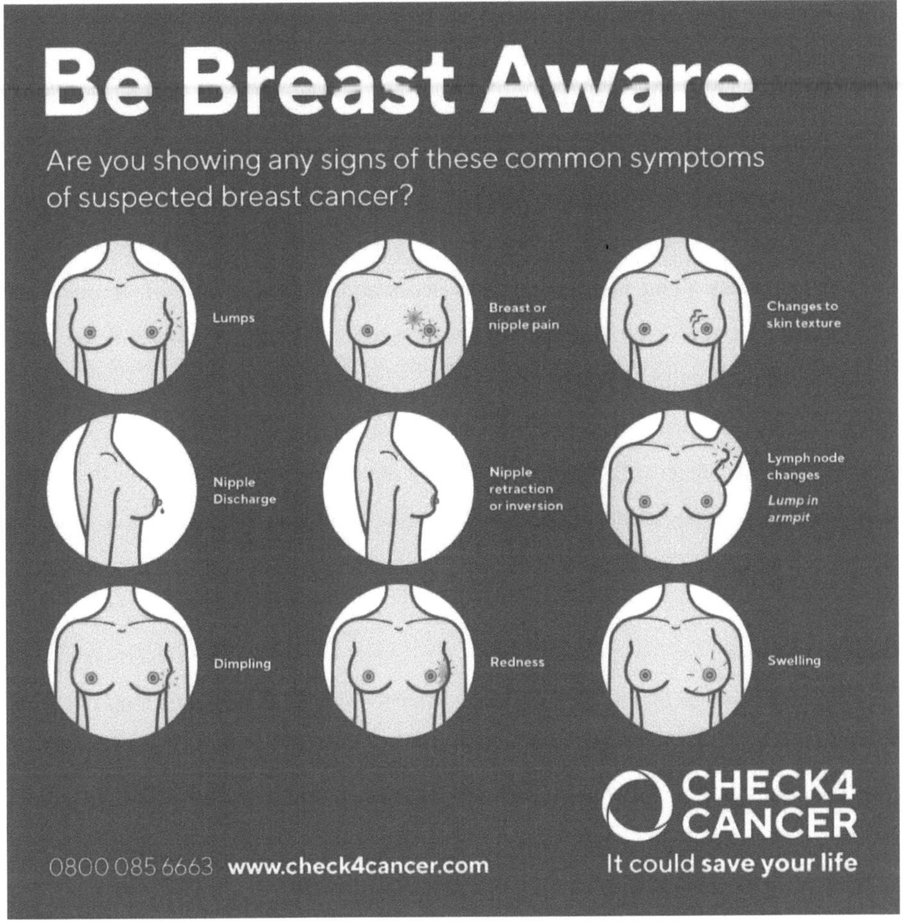

Figure 5. Breast Cancer Risk Factors & Symptoms

Screening and diagnosis

The use of conventional screening methods is recommended in patients who have any risk factors or symptoms. Among the diagnostic methods used to screen this cancer, the following tests can be mentioned.

- ✓ **Examination of the rectum:** In this examination, the doctor examines the blood of the rectum with a finger to check for any cases and if there are substances in the rectum, they should be examined for blood.

- ✓ **Proctoscopy:** In this method, it is observed directly into the rectum and lower parts of the large intestine through special devices. Half of all cancers can be diagnosed this way. In this method, the patient may feel pressure, but will not feel pain.

- ✓ **Colonoscopy:** Through this method, it is possible to observe the colon and rectum with special tools. In this case, too, the person will not feel pain. If there is any mass along these areas, it is necessary to remove part of the mass to examine under a microscope for the presence of tissue or cancer cells. This procedure is called a biopsy.

Prognosis and treatment of colorectal cancer depends on the stage of the disease, meaning that the cancer cells have affected only the lining of the intestine or the entire wall, and the general health of the patient. After treatment, a blood test is done to measure an antigen in the blood and an x-ray is done to see if the cancer has come back.

Stages of cancer

Recurrence of cancer means its recurrence after treatment. Recurrence may occur in the large intestine or other parts of the body, such as the liver or lungs. If the recurrence is an infection of only one area of the body, surgery should be performed, but if more than one area is involved and the cancer has spread to different parts of the body, other methods such as chemotherapy or radiotherapy may be used.

Treatment methods

There are generally three treatments for colon cancer, including surgery, radiation therapy, and chemotherapy. There is another method of treatment in which biological methods are used for treatment. Of course, the use of these methods is limited to clinical studies.

1- Surgery: Surgery is the most common treatment in all stages of cancer. This method is done in different ways and depending on the doctor's opinion and the stage of the cancer, the surgical methods are different.

- ✓ **Side effects of surgery:** Side effects of surgery depend on the location of the tumor and the type of surgery. The patient usually feels discomfort in the first few days after surgery, but the pain can usually be controlled with medication. The recovery time after surgery varies from patient to patient.

2- Radiation therapy: In this method, high energy X-rays are used to kill cancer cells and reduce the size of the tumor. Radiation can be produced outside the body by special machines or inside the body through materials that produce radiation. Radiation therapy is performed alone or in combination with surgery and chemotherapy.

- ✓ **Side effects of radiation therapy:** The most common side effects of radiation therapy include fatigue, skin reaction at the site of radiation to the skin, and loss of appetite. In addition, it may reduce the number of white blood cells that protect the body against infections. Some of these complications are controllable and treatable, and in many cases these complications are not permanent.

3- Chemotherapy: This method of drugs is used to kill cancer cells. Most anticancer drugs are given as an internal injection into the body or intramuscularly, but others can be taken orally. Chemotherapy is a systemic treatment in which the drug travels through the bloodstream to any part of the body to kill cancer cells. In this method, drugs are prescribed periodically. That is, the treatment period continues with a rest period, after which the treatment period begins again. If liver cancer cells are involved, the drug can be injected directly into the arteries that feed the liver. After the surgeon removes all the cancer cells and tissue through surgery, a course of chemotherapy is given to kill the remaining cancer cells, if any.

✓ **Side effects of chemotherapy:** Chemotherapy drugs usually target cells with high proliferation rates. Because in the body, in addition to cancer cells, tissues such as blood cells, gastrointestinal epithelium, and hair follicle cells also have a high rate of proliferation, these tissues may also be targeted by chemotherapy drugs. As a result, side effects include infections, fatigue, temporary hair loss, mouth sores, or other symptoms. One of the most important side effects of chemotherapy drugs is the general reduction of blood cells. Because chemotherapy drugs severely affect the bone marrow, it can cause anemia (reduced energy to do things), decrease blood platelets (bleeding), or decrease white blood cells (increased susceptibility to infections). Not everyone who uses this treatment usually has all of these symptoms. In addition, during the rest period and after stopping treatment, all these symptoms disappear.

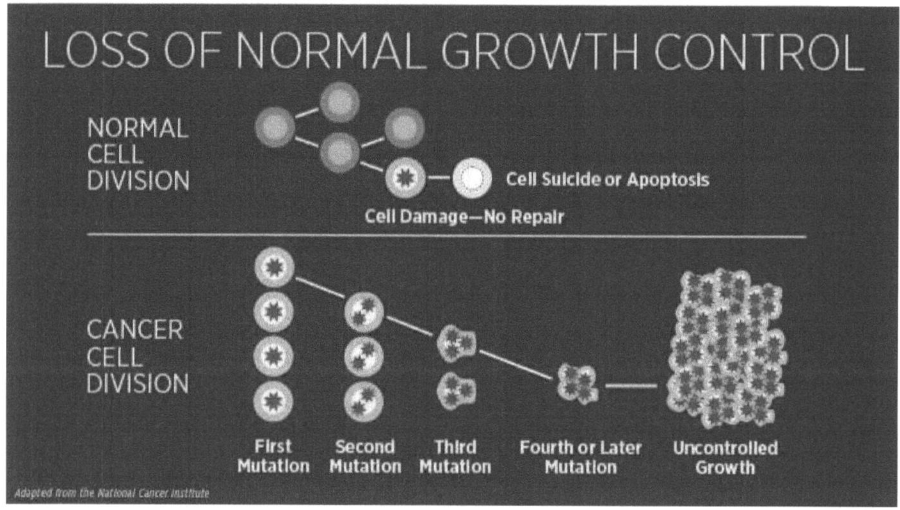

Figure 6. What Is Cancer? American Association for Cancer Research (AACR)

Biological therapies: In this method, the body alone fights against cancers. This method uses materials that are made by the body or in laboratories to direct, strengthen and maintain the body's natural defense mechanisms against disease. Another name for this method is immunotherapy.

Cervical Cancer

What is cervical cancer?

Cervical cancer is one of the most common cancers in women in which cancer cells inside the uterus begin to grow and multiply. The cervix is the entrance to the uterus and is where the uterus connects to the vagina. Cervical cancer grows slowly. Before the cancer cells appear in the cervix, the uterine tissue begins to make changes that do not look normal. These cells can be detected by Pap smear test. After these initial changes, the cancer cells begin to grow and grow deep into the surrounding tissues.

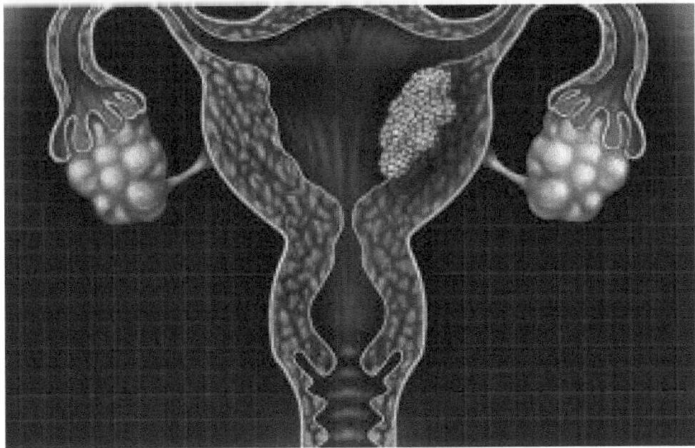

Figure 7. Cervical Cancer

If this cancer is identified and treated early, this type of cancer will be curable. In pre-invasive cancers, the 5-year survival rate is 100 percent, and in the early stages of invasive cancer, it will be 91 percent. In general, in all stages, in combination, this rate is 70%. Although the causes of this cancer are not fully understood, scientists have found out how this cancer grows and develops. Before the cancer cells grow, the cervical tissue begins to change, which is different from normal tissue. These changes happen slowly over several years, but sometimes they change very quickly. If abnormal precancerous cells form on the cervix, they are usually diagnosed when a woman has a Pap smear. Sometimes these cells disappear without treatment, but in most cases, there is a need for treatment. If the cells do not disappear on their own and are not treated, the cancer cells will start to grow and penetrate deep into the cervical tissue and surrounding tissues. The most common type of cervical cancer is squamous cell carcinoma.

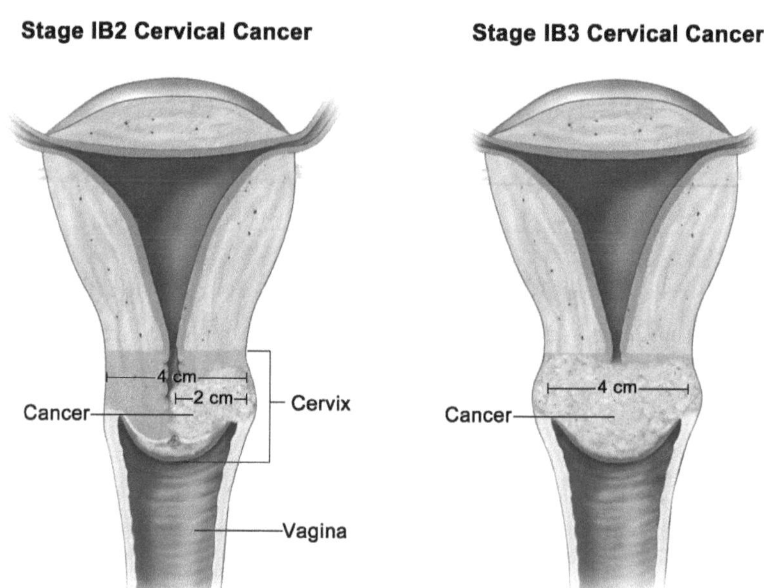

Figure 8. Cervical Cancer Treatment

Risk factors and prevention

The best way to prevent cervical cancer is to get an early Pap smear to screen for abnormal cervical cancer cells. If abnormal cells are found, they must be treated before the cancer cells can form. Women should have this test annually from the age of 18 until the end of their lives. In general, there are factors in general health that affect the risk of developing this type. Women who are at higher risk should see a doctor for a Pap smear.

Risk factors that affect the incidence of cervical cancer include the following:

Wart virus infection: Being infected with this virus, which is a sexually transmitted disease, increases your chances of getting cervical cancer.

Infection with AIDS: Infection with the AIDS virus suppresses the immune system and as a result the body loses the ability to fight precancerous and cancerous cells just like infections.

Smoking: Women who smoke are twice as likely to get it as non-smokers. Because cigarette smoke creates substances that damage normal cells in the cervix.

Symptoms and diagnosis

This type of cancer usually does not cause any symptoms. Therefore, routine screening tests are very important to look for any abnormal cervical tissue. Women who have symptoms such as abnormal discharge, unusual bleeding compared to menstrual bleeding, and vaginal discharge and pain during intercourse should see a doctor immediately. These symptoms may be secondary to infections or other problems, but they can sometimes occur when abnormal cells turn into primary cancer cells. Pap smear is a common test for screening abnormal cells in the precancerous stages. In this test, a doctor used a simple tool to take a sample of cervical tissue and inside it. The person may feel pressure during the test, but this test will usually not be painful. After sampling, the cells are sent to a laboratory for evaluation. If the test shows abnormal cells, the doctor may need to look directly at the cervical tissue through a special instrument called a colposcope. Sometimes cervical tissue sampling may be done to examine the specimen under a microscope and to assess the presence of cancer cells inside the tissue. This procedure is called a biopsy. If the required sample is small, this operation can also be done in the doctor's office, but if a larger sample is needed. For example, if a conical specimen is required, this operation should be performed in a hospital. The prognosis (chance of recovery) and the choice of treatment depend on the stage of the cancer (has the cancer only affected the cervical tissue or has it affected other tissues as well?) And the patient's general health status. In order to assess the spread of cancer cells to other tissues, other tests may be needed and based on the results of the tests, the cancer is divided into different stages.

Recurrence: Recurrence of cancer means its recurrence after treatment. Recurrence may occur in the cervix or other parts of the body. If recurrence of pelvic cancer occurs, one of the treatments is to use chemotherapy to relieve the symptoms of cancer. If recurrence occurs outside the pelvis, the patient may choose to undergo chemotherapy that is undergoing clinical trials.

Types of treatments and side effects

There are basically three treatments, including surgery, chemotherapy and radiation therapy. Because it is very difficult to kill cancer cells without damaging normal tissue, side effects are inevitable.

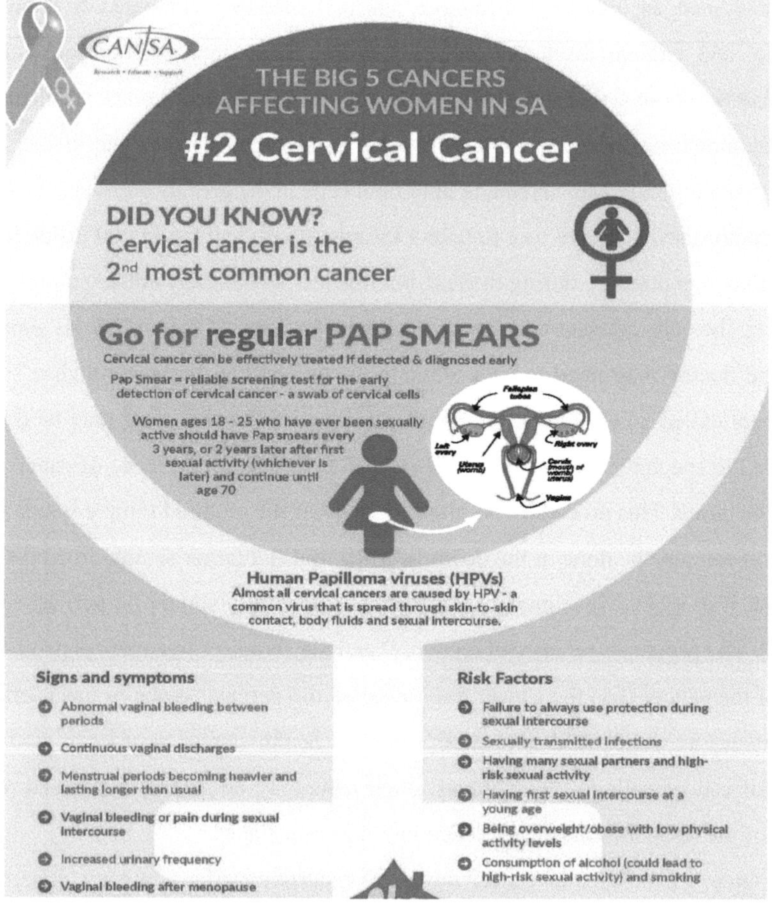

Figure 9. Cervical Cancer

1- Surgery: There are several surgical methods for the treatment of this type of cancer, the choice of each of which is up to the doctor.

- ✓ **Side effects:** Side effects vary depending on the location of the tumor and the type of operation and other factors. Although the person is upset in the first few days after surgery, the pain can be controlled with different medications. The recovery time also varies from person to person.

2- Radiation therapy: In this method, X-rays are used to kill cancer cells and reduce the size of the tumor. The beam is produced externally by special machines or internally by implanting special radioactive materials inside the body and near the tumor.

- ✓ **Side effects:** The most common side effects of this method are fatigue of skin reactions (in the form of skin rash and redness) at the site of radiation exposure, loss of appetite. If the pelvis is irradiated, the vagina may become narrow. Premature menopause, urinary disorders and low white blood cells may also occur. Of course, these side effects can be controlled and in many cases are not permanent.

3- Chemotherapy: In this method, drugs are used to kill cancer cells. Many chemotherapy drugs are given intravenously or intramuscularly. But their oral form is also available. This treatment is a systemic method. Because the drug is spread throughout the body through the blood and wherever there is a cancer cell, it kills it. This treatment is usually prescribed periodically. That is, after the treatment period, a period of rest is given and then the treatment period starts again.

- ✓ **Side effects:** Because these drugs also target tissues that have a high rate of proliferation. Therefore, blood cells, gastrointestinal lining, and hair follicle cells are also involved. Complications such as infection, fatigue, temporary hair loss, oral and vaginal ulcers, changes in the menstrual cycle and infertility may also occur. Of course, not all of these side effects occur in all cases, and they usually go away during the rest period or after stopping treatment. In addition, there are special medications and treatments to control and reduce these side effects.

Prostate Cancer

Prostate cancer is the second most common cause of cancer death in men, but can be successfully treated if diagnosed early. Symptoms of this cancer include vague pelvic pain, frequent urination, and other urinary disorders such as inability to urinate, pain during urination, poor urinary flow, blood in the urine and semen, and painful ejaculation. In addition to the above, the presence of pain in the back, pelvis and upper extremities, loss of appetite and weight, and persistent bone pain are other symptoms of this type of cancer.

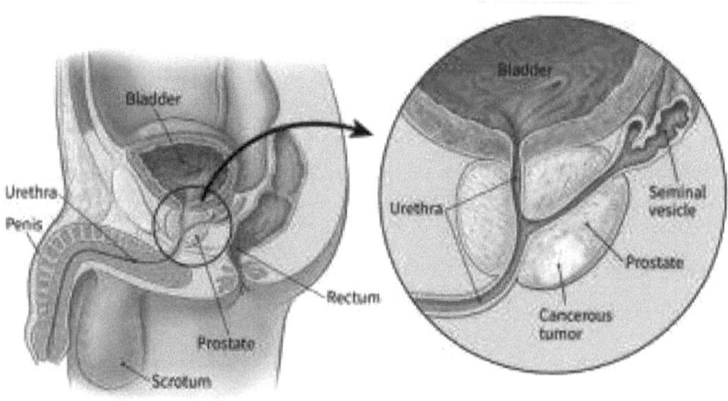

Figure 10. What Is Prostate Cancer?

It is recommended that men over the age of 40 usually have a rectal examination with a finger by themselves or a doctor to detect the size of the prostate, its abnormal shape, or the presence of any lumps in the prostate. It is also recommended that men over the age of 50 have an annual rectal exam with a specific test to measure prostate-specific antigen. This test is a blood test that measures the level of antigen. This antigen enters the bloodstream normally and regularly, but increases if the prostate gland becomes cancerous. In addition, a biopsy can be done using special tools. A specialist doctor may take 14 biopsies of the prostate gland at the same time. The samples are then examined by a pathologist to determine if the tissue has become cancerous and what stage it is at if it has become cancerous, and if cancer is diagnosed, there are several treatments that can kill the cancer cells. These methods can be combined with radiation therapy, in which cancer cells are killed using radiation. Another treatment is hormone therapy, especially when the cancer is in its early stages. This method uses drugs that reduce blood testosterone. This treatment regimen is given in the early stages of cancer, during which it is determined whether the cancer will enter a phase of failure or not. The latest treatment is to remove the prostate gland through surgery, which itself has different types.

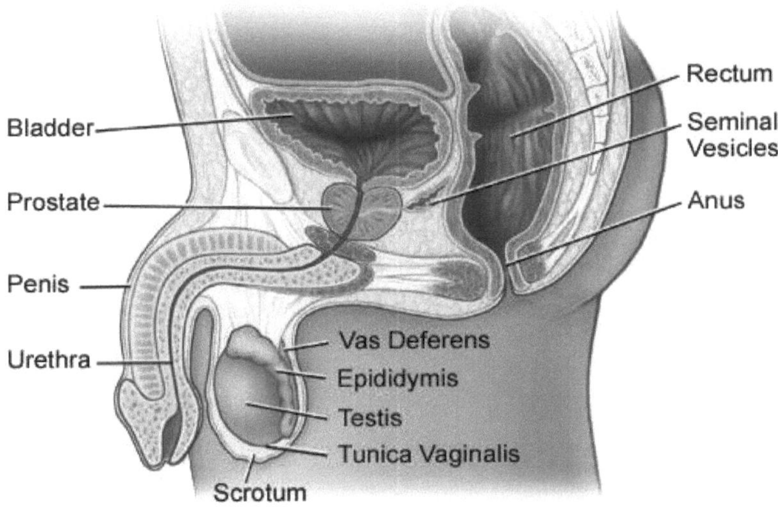

Figure 11. What is Prostate Cancer? Causes, Risks, Symptoms, Diagnosis, Treatment

Causes of natural garlic and diagnosis of prostate cancer

As mentioned, this cancer is the second leading cause of cancer death in men, but if diagnosed early and in the early stages, it can be treated significantly and effectively.

What is a prostate?

This organ is located as a small gland under the bladder and covers the upper part of the urethra. This gland is located in front of the rectum and its dorsal surface can be felt through examination of the rectum. (Anal examination) The function of this gland is to make a fluid that makes up part of the semen. This gland leads to a number of disorders in men, including the size of this gland, its inflammation and cancer.

What is prostate cancer?

Due to its high incidence, this cancer is one of the most common health problems. This type of cancer is different from other cancers in that a significant percentage of men with it have asymptomatic forms. This type of cancer usually does not cause any symptoms and does not spread outside the prostate gland. Sometimes the cancer is small and grows slowly and is less dangerous for the patient.

What are the risk factors for prostate cancer?

This type of secondary cancer appears to be caused by a variety of causes. The cancer usually affects the elderly and rarely occurs before the age of 40, but after that age the incidence increases significantly. Statistics worldwide show the third most common cancer and the sixth death from cancer in men for this cancer. Genetic causes and diet and race appear to be involved. Men with a family history of this cancer. They will have a better chance of getting it. Eating certain diets may reduce your chances of getting this cancer. Like foods rich in lycopene, selenium and vitamin E, cooked tomatoes are a source of carotenoid lycopene. These compounds are antioxidant compounds that protect cells against cancer. Numerous studies have shown that using these compounds in large quantities can reduce the chances of developing this cancer. Selenium intake can also reduce the chances of developing this cancer. The incidence of this cancer in some men appears to be secondary to reduced exposure to the sun and the body's ability to make this vitamin.

What are the signs and symptoms of prostate cancer?

In the early stages of this cancer there are no symptoms and in other cases the symptoms include vague pelvic pain, frequent urination, other administrative disorders such as inability to urinate, pain or burning urination, decreased urine flow, blood in the urine or semen, painful ejaculation, Pain in the lower back and upper legs is a decrease in appetite or weight and permanent bone pain.

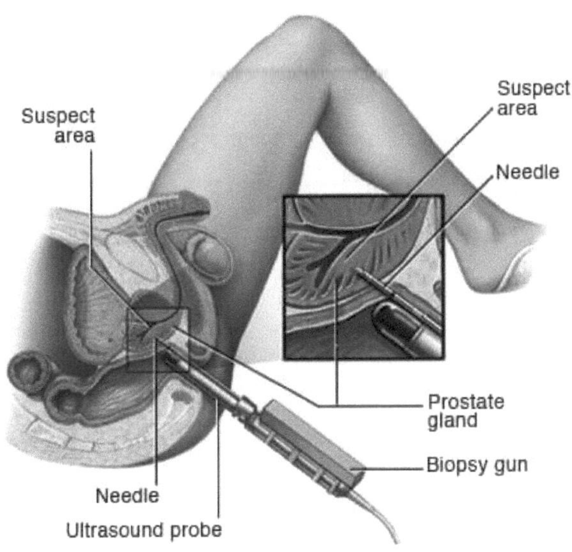

Figure 12. Prostate cancer - Diagnosis and treatment

Prostate cancer screening

Direct rectal examination and measurement of prostate-specific antigen are currently used to diagnose prostate cancer. The age of onset of these screening methods is not known exactly, but most experts believe that these two methods should be performed for cancer screening over the age of 50 years. But in those who are more likely to be infected, such as those with a positive family history, screening should be done at a younger age, 40 years.

Finger examination of the rectum

To do this, examine the face while the patient is prostrating or lying on his side Takes. In order to examine, the doctor inserts his finger into the rectum of the person being examined while wearing gloves, and examines the prostate for size, consistency, or the presence of any other mass inside the rectum. Since this method alone is not enough to diagnose prostate cancer, specific prostate measurements should also be used. This test is performed in a laboratory or hospital and does not require many tools. A blood sample is taken from the patient and the sample will be sent to the laboratory for testing. Normally, the amount of this antigen is very low, but in some cases, it increases, which is a sign of non-cancerous prostate cancer or prostate cancer. It is now recommended that both be performed together in order to diagnose prostate cancer early and early. Of course, it should be noted that the presence of any abnormalities in the above two methods does not necessarily mean cancer and can be secondary to the benign size of the prostate.

Brain tumors (Brain Cancers)

What are brain tumors?

The brain is responsible for controlling memory, learning, feeling and emotion. In addition, this organ monitors other parts of the body such as muscles, organs and arteries. Brain cancer is a disease in which cancer cells inside the brain tissue begin to grow and multiply. This article examines brain cancers that originate in the brain tissue itself. In most cases, cancers that develop in the brain are secondary to the spread of cancer from other parts of the body to this area. This type of diffusion is called metastasis. If a person has the following symptoms, he should see a doctor. Persistent headache, vomiting or difficulty walking or talking. After confirming the symptoms, the patient must have a CT scan or MRI. In most cases, it is necessary to determine surgically whether or not there is a brain tumor, and if so, to determine its type. If a brain tumor is confirmed, the type and stage of the tumor are determined using special methods. Because these factors are influential in deciding how to treat and treat cancer.

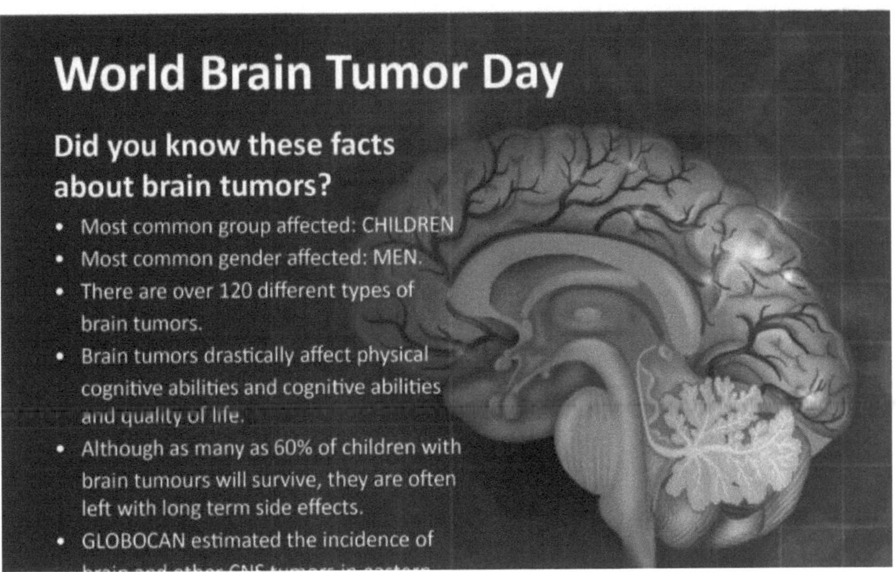

Figure 13. World Brain Tumor Day

Recurrence of brain tumors

Tumor recurrence means the growth of two cancers after treatment. Tumor recurrence can occur in the brain itself or in other parts of the body. In these cases, treatment depends on the type of tumor and how it is initially treated.

Treatment methods

In general, three treatments are used to treat brain cancers, including surgery, radiation therapy, and chemotherapy.

1- Surgery: Surgery is the most common treatment for brain tumors. In order to reach the tumor, the surgeon first removes a piece of skull bone to reach the brain. This operation is called a craniotomy. After the doctor removes the cancerous tissue, he or she places the removed piece in place or uses a piece of metal instead. The surgeon tries to remove all the cancerous tissue as much as possible, but it is not clear exactly whether the entire cancerous tissue has been removed or not. Because the cancer invades some parts of the brain tissue in such a way that the removal of those areas must be accompanied by the removal of part of the healthy brain tissue.

2- Radiation therapy: In this method, high-energy rays are used to cause damage to cancer cells and stop their growth and proliferation. This treatment is topical and only the area that has been irradiated is treated. Radiation can be emitted from an external source (radiation generating machines) or from an internal source (using implants in the body near the tumor).

3- Chemotherapy: In this method, special drugs are used to kill cancer cells. Most anticancer drugs are given intravenously or intramuscularly, but some are taken orally. This treatment is a systemic method, which means that the drug is distributed throughout the body through the bloodstream and destroys cancer cells anywhere in the body. The use of this method is periodic and after the treatment period, a period of rest is given and then another course of treatment is started again.

Side effects of treatment methods

The various treatments used to treat cancers have their own side effects. Because in all these methods, in addition to cancerous tissue, healthy tissue is also damaged in some areas. The type and extent of side effects vary depending on the treatment method, duration of use and amount.

Surgery: The side effects of surgery depend on the location and type of tumor. Although patients feel uncomfortable during the first few days after surgery, the pain can be controlled with medication. The recovery period after surgery varies from person to person. Long-term neurological disorders may develop after brain surgery.

Chemotherapy: This method usually targets cancer cells with a high rate of proliferation, but in addition to cancer cells, other healthy tissues in the body that have a high rate of proliferation, such as blood cells, gastrointestinal cells and hair follicle cells are also affected. These medications are prescribed and side effects such as infections, fatigue, temporary hair loss and mouth ulcers may occur. However, it should be noted that not all patients develop all of these complications, and these complications resolve during the rest period and after cessation of treatment. There are certain medications and treatments that can control or reduce these symptoms. Blood cell depletion is one of the most important side effects of many chemotherapy drugs. Because these drugs severely affect the bone marrow, where blood cells are made, they can lead to complications such as anemia (the patient may have less energy to do things, and if the anemia is severe, they may need Blood transfusions (decrease in platelets (the patient may simply bleed and need platelets if severe) and antibodies (the patient may be more susceptible to infections).

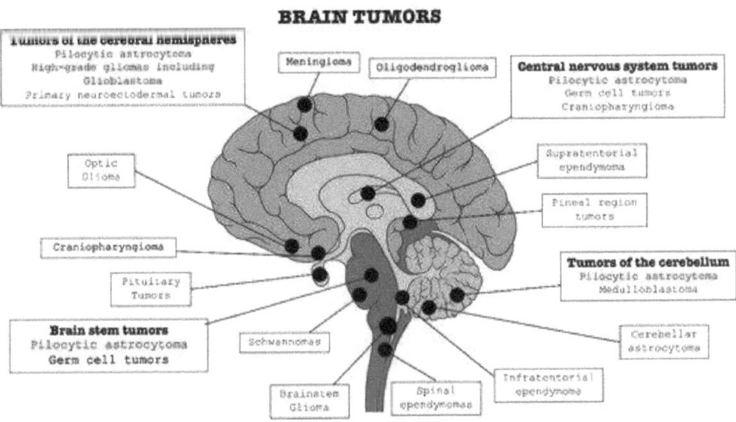

Figure 14. Role of Fibroblast Growth Factors Receptors (FGFRs) in Brain Tumors

Radiation therapy: The most common side effects of this method are fatigue. Skin reactions at the site of radiation exposure (in the form of skin rashes and redness) also reduce the appetite of white blood cells, which help the body fight infections. Most of these complications are controllable and treatable, and many are temporary.

During cancer treatment, the patient feels loss of appetite and difficulty eating. In addition, other side effects such as nausea, vomiting and mouth ulcers are more common. In some people, the taste of food also changes. Proper nutrition means getting enough calories and protein to prevent weight loss and maintain body strength. Patients who eat well during treatment will feel better and have more energy, as well as a greater ability to tolerate the side effects of treatment methods.

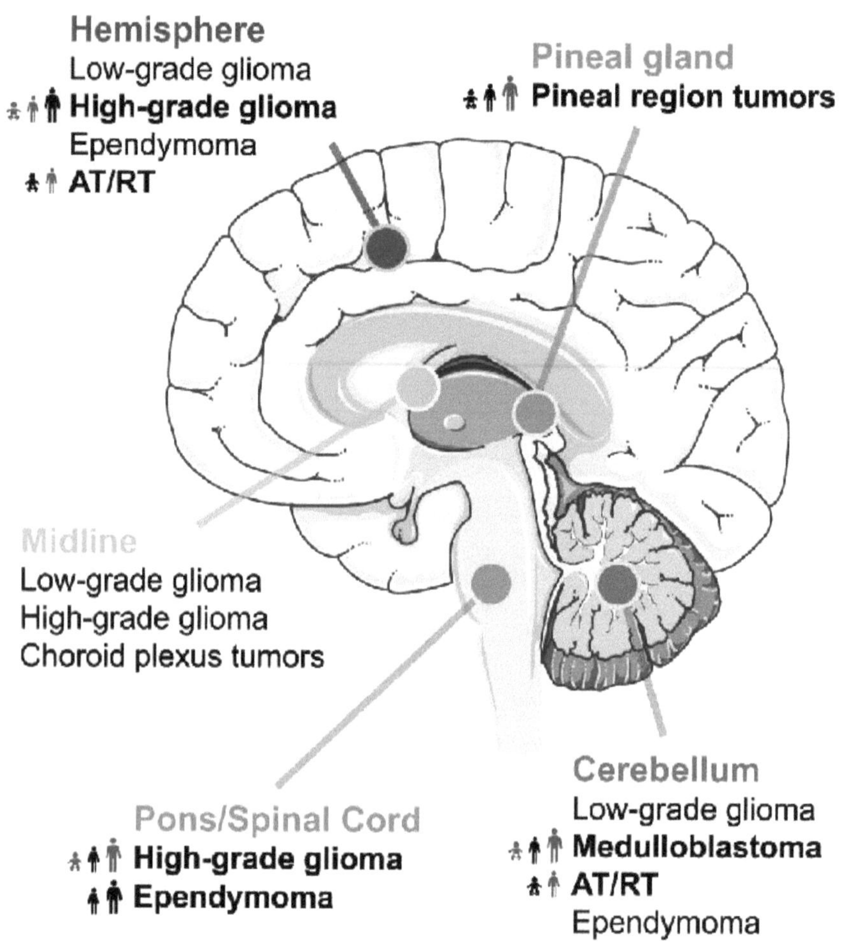

Figure 15. Location of common brain tumors. Tumor entities

Non-melanoma skin cancers

What is non-melanoma skin cancer?

Skin cancer is a disease in which cancer cells form in the outermost layers of the skin. The skin has several main layers and different types of cells. The top layer of skin is called the epidermis, and there are several types of cells that can become cancerous in this layer, including basal cells, squamous cells, and melanocytes (pigment cells). The most common skin cancer is basal cell carcinoma. Squamous cell carcinoma, both of which are called non-melanoma skin cancers. Melanoma is a type of skin cancer in which melanoma develops into cancer cells. This form is less common but very dangerous and more difficult to treat than the previous two types. Therefore, it is examined separately. The incidence of non-melanoma skin cancer is increasing in the United States, and both basal cell and squamous cell carcinomas are more common in people with fair skin, especially those with light hair and eyes who do not tan easily. Non-melanoma skin cancer is rare in black people. Basal cell carcinoma is also the most common type of non-melanoma skin cancer and accounts for more than 90% of skin cancers. This cancer is more common in areas of the skin that are exposed to sunlight. The cancer appears as a small bump with a glossy border on the head, neck, and hands. Sometimes it is wide, which is mostly on the trunk. This type of cancer is difficult to detect and grows very slowly (it may take months or years for the tumor to reach a centimeter in diameter) and is excellent for treatment. If the treatment is done correctly, the 5-year survival rate will be more than 99%. Basal cell carcinoma usually does not spread to other parts of the body and usually spreads to surrounding areas. Sometimes it may extend deep into the skin and into the bones, which can lead to significant local damage. In addition, non-melanoma skin cancers increase a person's chances of developing other types of cancer. Squamous cell carcinoma also occurs in areas of the body that are exposed to sunlight, such as the nose, forehead, lower lip, and hands. It also occurs in other areas of the body that have been burned, exposed to chemicals, or treated with radiation. This type of cancer usually appears as a hard red spot or with a scab. In a small number of cases, the cancer spreads to other parts of the body. The 5-year survival rate for this type of cancer is more than 95%.

Causes and risk factors

The sun's ultraviolet rays: The main cause of skin cancers is the sun's ultraviolet rays. Excessive and constant exposure to sunlight can lead to skin cancer. Due to the depletion of the ozone layer in the Earth's atmosphere, the amount of ultraviolet radiation reaching the Earth has increased compared to 50 to 100 years ago, and as a result, the incidence of skin cancer has increased. The ozone layer as a filter reduces the amount of ultraviolet radiation that reaches the earth. Therefore, by reducing the effect of this layer, the amount of radiation that reaches the earth's surface is more. The number of rays that reach a person from the sun varies depending on their lifestyle and geographical location. People who are exposed to sunlight for more hours of the day are more likely to get these types of cancers. In addition, people who live at higher altitudes (because the air is lower than sea level) or at higher altitudes near the equator (closer to the sun) may be more likely to be infected. In areas where the weather is cloudy most days, the residents of these areas may be exposed to 50% of the sun's ultraviolet rays. Two other factors involved in the development of these cancers include heredity or the presence of numerous abnormal moles on the skin.

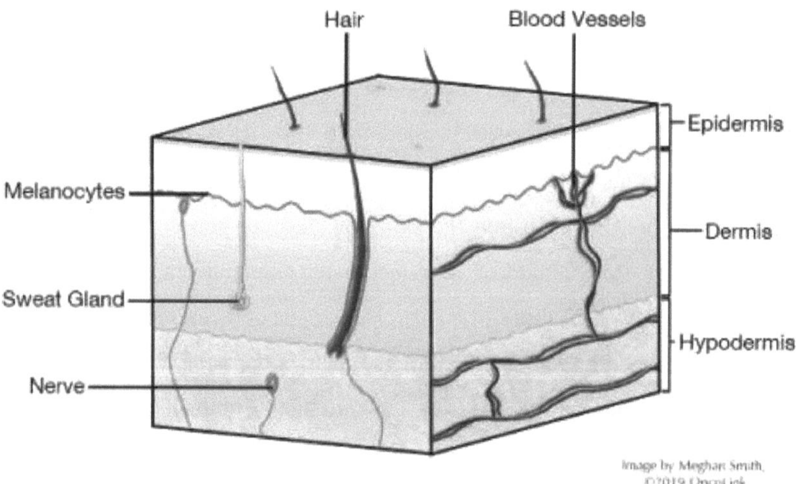

Figure 16. All about Non-Melanoma Skin Cancers

Heredity: People with a family history of skin cancers are more likely to develop these types of cancers. Whites and those living in northern Europe are also more sensitive.

Existence of multiple and abnormal moles: People who have a lot of these types of moles have a slightly higher chance of getting them.

Treatment methods

In general, three treatments are used to treat these cancers, including surgery, chemotherapy, and radiation therapy. Biological therapies and photodynamic therapies are also currently being studied. The treatment of choice varies according to the location and extent of the cancer and the patient's health status.

1- **Surgery:** Surgery is the most common treatment for skin cancers and in about 90% of cases, this treatment has been used. One of the side effects of this method is that the operation site remains on the skin. Therefore, depending on the size of the cancer, some skin may be removed from another part of the body and placed in the operating environment. This operation is called a skin graft.

2- **Radiation therapy:** In this method, X-rays are used to kill cancer cells and reduce the size of the cancer. In this method, the required radiation is generated by an external machine.

3- **Chemotherapy:** In this method, drugs are used to kill cancer cells. In this method, the drug is used as a cream or lotion, which is called dermal dermal chemistry. In addition, the drug can be used as a pill or intramuscular or intravenous injection. This method is a kind of systemic method. Because the drug is distributed through the bloodstream to different parts of the body. The use of systemic therapies for the treatment of skin cancers is limited to clinical studies.

4- **Biological methods:** In this method, the body's immune system is used to fight cancer. This method is also within the scope of clinical studies. In this method, materials made by the body or in the laboratory are used to strengthen the body's natural defense against diseases. Another name for this method is immunotherapy.

5- Photodynamic therapies: In this method, specific wavelengths and special chemicals are used to kill cancer cells.

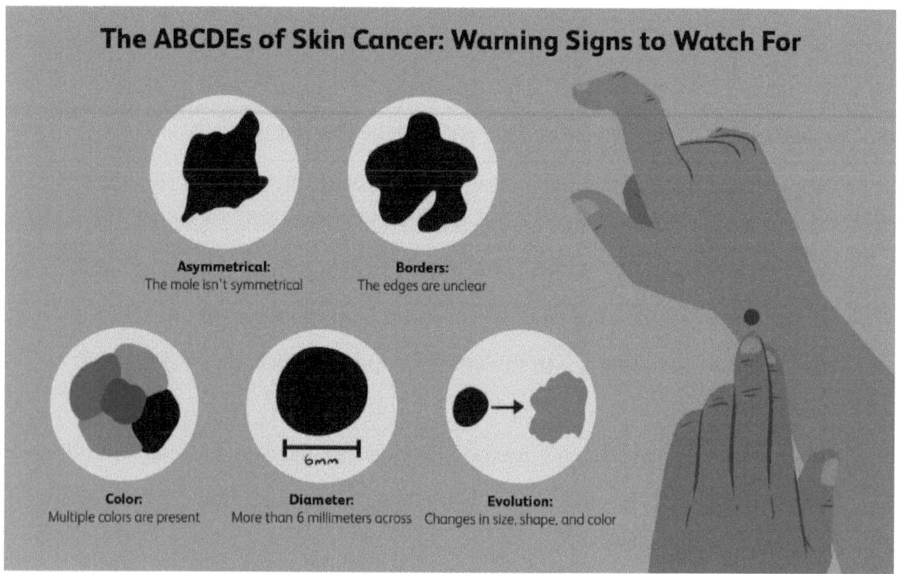

Figure 17. What Is Nonmelanoma Skin Cancer?

General examination of leukemias

What is leukemia?

Leukemia means cancer of the blood cells. Usually, among the blood types, white blood cells are more prone to cancer. Cancer cells are different from normal blood cells and have lost their normal function. Blood cancers are divided into two categories, each of which manifests itself in both acute and chronic forms. In acute leukemia, there are large numbers of primary and immature cells called blasts in the bloodstream, which are usually very immature and lack normal function. The rate of proliferation of these cells is very high and the disease spreads rapidly. Chronic leukemia also has blast cells, but these cells are more mature and able to perform some of their functions. In this case, the cells grow more slowly and the progression of the disease is slower.

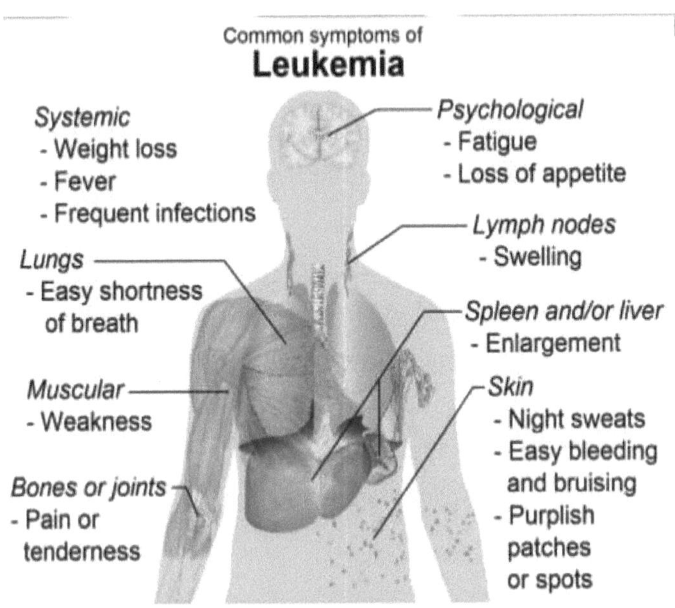

Figure 18. Leukemia

What are the symptoms of leukemia?

The following are some of the most common symptoms of leukemia, but each person may have other symptoms. Increased incidence of infections and fever, anemia and related symptoms including pale skin, fatigue and weakness, bleeding, bruising and hemorrhage, fever and chills, loss of appetite, weight loss, swollen lymph nodes, large and painful liver and spleen the red spots are full of skin, swelling and bleeding from the gums, sweating and pain in the bones and joints. In addition, acute leukemia can lead to headaches, vomiting, dizziness, lack of muscle control, seizures, swollen testicles, and sores in the eyes or on the skin. Chronic leukemia can also affect the skin, central nervous system, gastrointestinal tract, kidneys and testicles. Other blood disorders or certain medications may cause similar symptoms. Therefore, if you see these symptoms, see your doctor.

How is leukemia diagnosed?

In addition to obtaining a complete history and performing the necessary examinations, diagnostic methods for different types of leukemias include the following:

- ✓ Examination and evaluation of enlarged liver, spleen, lymph nodes behind the elbow, hip and neck.
- ✓ Performing blood tests and other necessary tests.
- ✓ Blood tests to assess the number of immature blood cells (blasts).
- ✓ Bone marrow sampling.
- ✓ Sampling of lumbar fluid.
- ✓ Imaging methods such as photography, ultrasound and CT scan.

Treatment of acute and chronic cancers

The use of specific treatments for a patient is the responsibility of the physician and based on the age, general health and medical history of the patient, the extent of the disease, the patient's tolerance to specific drugs or treatments, expectations of the course of the disease and their opinion and preference Is sick.

Therapies include: chemotherapy, radiation therapy, bone marrow stem cell transplants, biological therapies, blood transfusions, and the use of drugs that prevent the destruction of other body systems affected by the spread of cancer.

Causes and risk factors

Causes and risk factors that increase the risk of leukemia include exposure to radiation, exposure to chemicals such as benzene, which are more common in the workplace, and the use of chemotherapy drugs for others. Cancers such as breast and ovarian cancer and radiation therapy were mentioned.

Nutrition and cancer prevention

In the past, nutrition was thought to have no effect on cancer, but today researchers have proven that a daily diet plays an important role in the development, prevention and treatment of various cancers. Our bodies need food more than anything else, and it can be said that one third of the cancers that lead to death are related to what we eat. Developments in people's eating habits, the expansion of urbanization and the increase in the consumption of prepared foods have increased the incidence of cancer. Some of the factors that contribute to cancer, such as heredity or environmental factors, are immutable, but if we cannot change our environmental factors, we can significantly reduce the risk of cancer by modifying and balancing dietary patterns. Causes of cancer vary from country to country. In urban and developed communities, overeating (ovrnutrition) and in poor communities' undernutrition cause cancer.

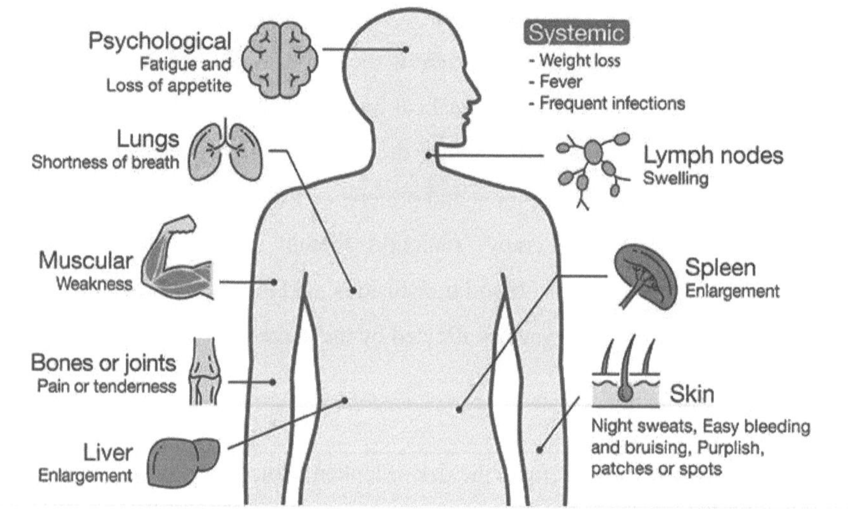

Figure 19. What Are Some of the Common Symptoms of Leukemia?

Fats

Fats and oils are important and controversial parts of a person's diet. There is a lot of question everywhere about which type of oil is suitable for consumption or which type of oil is more likely to cause disease, stroke or hyperlipidemia. As you probably know, there are many types of fats, such as saturated fats, including fats attached to meat and animal fats, which are solid at room temperature. Another type is unsaturated fats, such as olive oil, which is liquid at room temperature. The effect of fat consumption on the incidence of cancer is such that both the type and amount of fat consumed is important. If we consume too much fat, due to the high secretion of bile in the intestine to digest fats, part of it becomes apcholic acid, which plays an important role in causing colon cancer, and if by consuming too much cholesterol, the level of cholesterol Harmful blood or LDL increases the risk of cancer cell growth and the risk of clogged arteries.

Diet in Cancers

Diets were once thought to have no role in cancer deaths. Today, researchers have proven that people's daily diet plays an important role in the prevention, incidence and treatment of various cancers. Given the fact that humans are required to consume food on a daily basis, and due to the number and variety of cancers that are potentially related to diet, it can be said that about one-third of cancers that eventually lead to death are related to what we eat. Are communication. The impact of changes that have taken place in people's lifestyles and eating habits today cannot be ignored in causing such diseases. Undoubtedly, the susceptibility to cancer varies from person to person due to intrinsic and intrinsic differences, and in addition to hereditary characteristics, external factors also play a role in the development of cancers. Despite the growing prevalence of cancer around the world, we hear promising news about these diseases every day. If we cannot change our environmental factors or if we cannot overcome the environment and the threatening factors in it, but we can by modifying and balancing our eating patterns throughout life, the risk of cancer is significantly higher. Reduction. The study of populations that migrate from one region to another and as a result change their food culture has shown that these people are exposed to common cancers in the region due to changing dietary patterns and adopting a new pattern. There is a complex link between nutrition and diet and cancer. The food we eat can potentially contain carcinogens and precursors to cancer or, conversely, anti-cancer substances. The nature of cancer and its relationship with diet varies from region to region. Therefore, the same guidelines cannot be offered to all people. For example, in the industrialized countries of North America and Europe, there is a problem of over-nutrition in the incidence of cancer, and it seems that the high-fat and high-calorie diets common in these countries are associated with the increasing prevalence of various types of cancer. In contrast, the nature of the problem in developing countries is fundamentally different. What is problematic in these countries is the lack of nutrition (Under Nutrition) and the limited variety of dietary patterns. In such a model, the number of vitamins and nutrients that are essential for human health is insufficient. In addition, problems with food storage and storage significantly reduce the quality of food consumed by these people. Differences in the nature of the relationship between cancer and diet between different nations require that executive guidelines be proposed for each nation according to the characteristics of that population. The following is a summary of guidelines recommended by advocacy organizations, researchers, government agencies, and health agencies that are available to the general public.

1. Have a varied diet. Remember that the nutrients you need do not come from just one or two sources. Include all food groups in your daily diet: fruits, vegetables, grains, meat, dairy products, and so on.

2. Always keep the blood weight in balance. Obesity is a major cause of many diseases such as heart disease, vascular disease, hypertension, diabetes and the underlying cause of some cancers.

3. high fat intake. Foods's high in saturated fat and cholesterol. A high-fat diet can increase the risk of breast, prostate, colon and rectal cancers.

4. 4 - Increase the amount of starchy and fiber foods in your diet. It is easy to increase the amount of starch and fiber in the diet by eating fruits, vegetables, potatoes, seeds, breads and whole grains. A high-fiber diet reduces the risk of colon and rectal cancer.

5. Limit sweets. Diets that contain sweets and sugary foods are often high in fat, high in calories, and depleted of nutrients and minerals, which can lead to some cancers.

6. Reduce the salt in your diet as much as possible.

7. Stop consuming alcoholic beverages. Alcohol consumption can lead to cancers of the mouth, throat, esophagus and liver. The rate of cancer in alcoholics who smoke is several times higher.

What foods should we choose?

By choosing and including the following foods in your daily diet, you can reduce your risk of cancer.

1- Dietary fiber: Fiber is a part of plant cell structure that the human digestive system is not able to digest. Fiber helps move food through the gastrointestinal tract and remove waste products from the body, thereby maintaining the health of the gastrointestinal tract. Having a diet high in fiber and low in fat reduces the risk of colon and rectal cancer. The amount of fiber consumed in American societies is 11 grams per day, which according to the International Cancer Institute NCI, this amount should be increased to 20-30 grams per day. The NCI does not recommend consuming more than 35 grams of fiber per day. Because consuming more than this amount can have adverse effects. Use fiber-rich food sources instead of artificial fiber supplements to find the fiber you need. To do this, include a variety of breads, pastas and unrefined cereals in your diet. Try to reduce the consumption of products made from refined flours. Eat apples, peaches, pears and even potatoes with their skins and products made from refined flours. Baked beans and peas are excellent sources of fiber. High-fiber foods are usually low in fat.

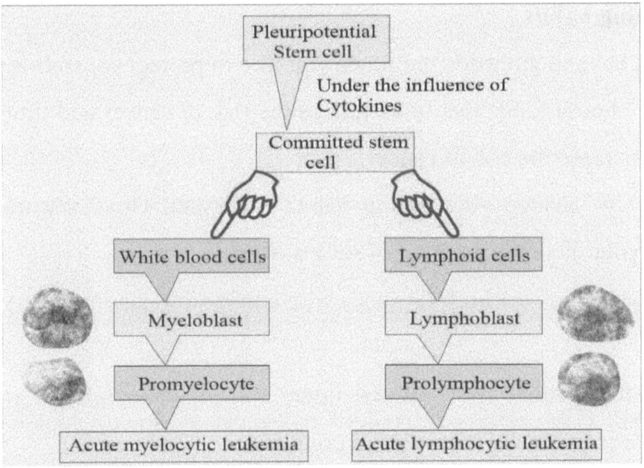

Figure 20. Acute Leukemias and their Diagnosis, Acute Myelocytic and Acute Lymphocytic Leukemia

2- Eat lean meats as much as possible in your daily diet. Before cooking the meat, remove all the visible fat and discard it, and if there is any fat left, remove it before eating. Increase fish consumption. Use white meat instead of red meat and remove the skin and fat before cooking.

3- Replace fried and high-fat snacks with fruits and vegetables.

4- Use low-fat dairy products instead of high-fat dairy products (whole milk, cream, buttermilk, etc.). This group of foods are good sources of protein, vitamins and minerals (minerals), especially calcium, which are useful for maintaining good health.

5- Eating foods rich in vitamin A, beta-carotene and vitamin C reduces the risk of cancer. There are many fruits and vegetables that contain the above ingredients. Try to include dark green, yellow and orange leafy vegetables and fruits, especially citrus fruits, in your daily diet.

6- Cabbage vegetables often reduce the risk of various cancers. These vegetables are good sources of fiber, vitamins and minerals. From this family, we can mention Chinese cabbage, broccoli, Brussels sprouts, kale, cauliflower and lunar cabbage.

Changing eating habits

1- You do not have to put aside the foods you like to protect yourself against cancer. Instead, try to choose foods that often reduce the risk of cancer and limit the number of foods that increase the risk of cancer.

2- Do not try to change your eating habits overnight. Gradually add fruits and vegetables to your diet over a period of several weeks.

3- Try to replace one of the high-fat foods with similar low-fat ones every time you go shopping.

4- Instead of foods made from refined flours and processed grains, such as white breads, use whole-grain and whole-grain products.

5- Use cooking methods that do not require the addition of oil. Such as grilling, steaming and boiling.

6- In methods such as grilling and grilling, avoid food contact with smoke. Contact of food with smoke can lead to the production of carcinogens in food.

7- Try to wrap the food in foil before grilling or frying and keep it away from the heat source to make the cooking time longer.

8- Try to set a diet plan for each day according to food labels and the amount of fat, calories and fiber in them.

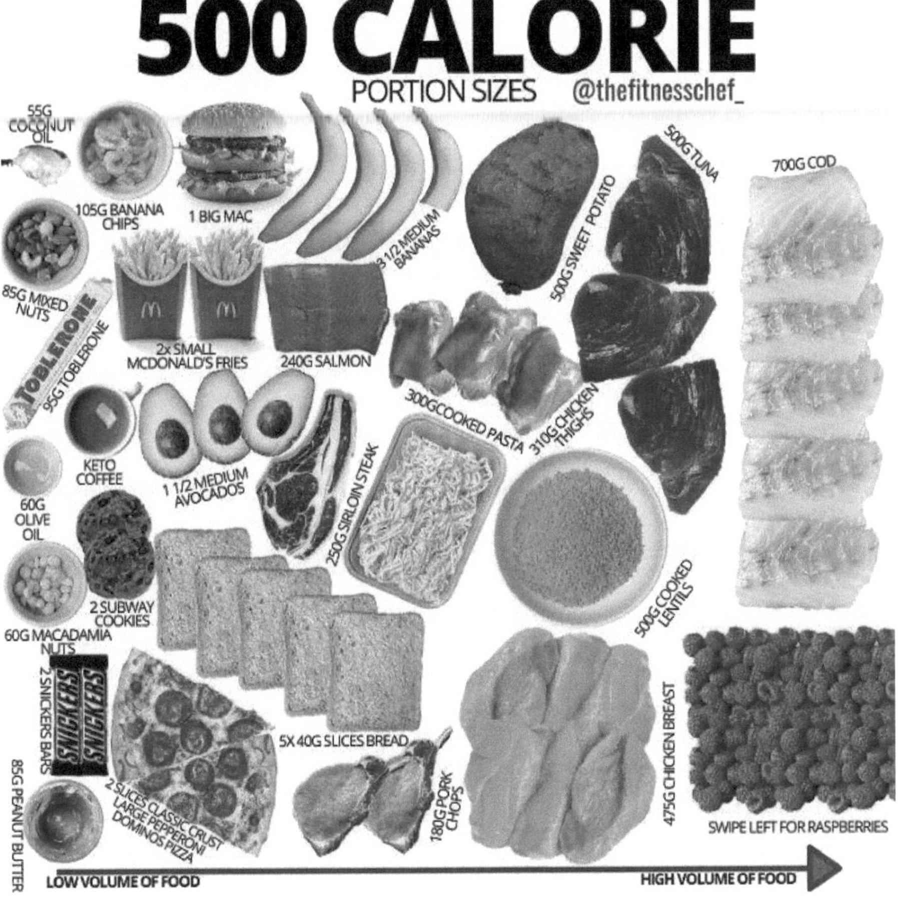

Figure 21. Food-Health-Charts

Chapter II

Stress in Breast Cancer Patients

Introduction

Breast cancer is the most important malignant tumor in women and is considered as the leader of young mothers' killers. Breast cancer has been identified in the United States as the first cancer death in women. The findings show that breast cancer patients suffered from psychological symptoms such as depression, anxiety, perceived stress, and feelings of helplessness. Part of this syndrome is due to the awareness of cancer and cognitive feedback and the other part is due to the side effects of common medical treatments such as mastectomy, chemotherapy, surgery, radiotherapy such as hair loss and body parts that symbolize being a woman and mother. Among the psychological symptoms, the amount of frustration and stress that a person perceives creates a special mental condition in which the person feels stagnant, helpless and uninterested in life. In this case, the person is severely inactive and does not have the power to adapt to changing living conditions and distances himself from the normal flow of life day by day. When people are in such a situation, they pay less attention to their public health, social relations, nutrition and other personal issues, and this in turn prepares the ground for the progression of cancer. Early diagnosis of breast cancer will be very important, because only in the early stages of the disease can be achieved with surgery and adjuvant therapies. As a result, the destruction of many families can be prevented. Special attention to this is a necessity of our society. Considering that comprehensive and accurate research in these cases has rarely been done in our country, it seems necessary to carefully examine the correlations of this disease. Cancer is a potentially dangerous disease that can cause many problems in employment, education or personal and social relationships and generally lead to economic and social disability for patients and their families. In addition to physical involvement, cancer causes stress and psychological distress in the patient. Cancer is one of the leading causes of death in the world today. More than 10 million new cases of cancer and more than 6 million deaths from cancer occur each year worldwide. It is estimated that by 2020 the world's population will reach 7.5 million, of which 15 million will develop cancer, of which 12 million will die from the disease. Cancer is currently the third leading cause of death in Iran, with 300,000 people dying of cancer each year in Iran. Although the cause of cancer is known to be multiple cell mutations, most mutations are due to interactions with the environment. Although the cause of cancer is considered to be multiple cell mutations, most mutations are due to interactions with the environment, and therefore more than half of them. It is preventable. Most people with cancer experience a period of stress that reduces their daily functioning. These psychiatric problems are so severe clinically that they even leave chemotherapy patients because of these problems. Given the importance of cancer and its high prevalence, it is necessary to identify the factors affecting it and control this phenomenon. The results of these studies can increase awareness of disease exacerbating factors and reduce the vulnerability of people with cancer by providing more information about the methods of control and treatment of this disease and by applying appropriate strategies.

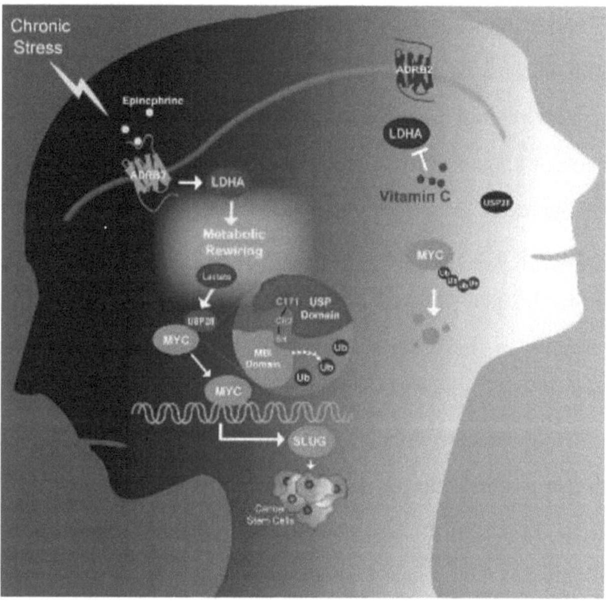

Figure 22. Mouse study reveals how chronic stress promotes breast cancer stem cells

Cancer is one of the most common chronic and contagious diseases. Cancer is caused by a mutation or abnormal activation of cell genes that control cell growth and mitosis, creating a competition between cancer cells and normal tissues for nutrients, and the cells have virtually all the nutrients available to the tissue. They absorb natural substances for the growth of their cells. As a result, the body's natural tissues gradually die from a lack of brain material. Despite significant advances in medical science, cancer is still one of the most important diseases of the present century and the second leading cause of death after cardiovascular disease. More than 7 million people worldwide are currently dying from cancer, and the number of new cases is projected to rise from 10 million to 15 million annually by 2020. All forms of cancer account for 9% of all deaths worldwide. Characteristics of cancer include fatigue, mental health problems, denial of the disease, impaired mental image due to changes in the function of organs and the duration of the disease. Cancer is the third leading cause of death in Iran. Breast cancer is the most common type of cancer in women and is the leading cause of death in women aged 35-45 years. Despite advances in the diagnosis and treatment of breast cancer, this disease is still the most common malignancy and the second leading cause of death due to satan in women. Is. Although the cause of cancer is considered to be multiple cell mutations, most mutations are the result of interactions with the environment, and therefore more than half of them are preventable.

In a review study, they concluded that external factors such as stress, depression and social support have a significant effect on the components of the immune system that affect the onset or course of cancer. In their view, the relationship between psychological factors and cancer is very complex and involves several biological, psychological and social systems.

In addition to the valuable findings of neurobiology and neurobiochemistry, attention to cultural and environmental factors of interpersonal aspects in terms of cognitive and emotional behavior is fully felt, there is a close relationship between psychological states and cancer. According to new research, stress is one of the most important causes of cancer in humans. Stress, anxiety, and stress exacerbate the risk of cancer in humans by affecting the immune system.

Every human being experiences stress throughout his life and it seems that this is an integral part of life and cannot be avoided. Stress is a physiological response to biological stressors (surgical and infectious terms) and psychological stressors such as anxiety and fear and social tensions. Perceived stress refers to a person's overall perception and interpretation of being affected by stressors. Different people perceive and interpret the same stressors in different ways, different factors can play a role in the formation of perceived stress and the person's interpretation of the amount of stress. In fact, people with breast cancer have high levels of stress.

In addition to stress, these people also have worries. From a cognitive point of view, anxiety is a chain of thoughts and mental images that has a negative and to some extent uncontrollable emotional theme. Some psychologists also consider anxiety to be an avoidant emotional response that in the short term reduces emotional distress, gains control, and prevents the manifestation of more intense negative emotions. But contrary to this protective function, when people have chronic problems such as cancer, anxiety can reduce long-term coping and increase anxiety, depression and other psychological problems, and naturally increase the problems of chronic patients such as cancer. A study aimed at investigating the relationship between breast cancer and life stress and personality as a trigger in the development of this cancer, showed that the number of high-risk events (stressful and worrying) in the group of patients with breast cancer it was significantly higher than the healthy group and this rate was 2.4 times higher than healthy individuals. Also, the severity of these events in the patient group was significantly higher than the healthy group. Therefore, there is a relationship between life events, high-risk life events and the severity of each of them with the incidence of breast cancer.

Also, people with cancer have little contact with others and acquaintances due to the nature of their disease, and this factor can cause them to feel lonely. In fact, the feeling of loneliness can be considered as a perceived inadequacy and weakness in interpersonal relationships, which is defined as the difference between the desired level and the existing level of social relations, and the greater the difference, the greater the feeling of loneliness. Some studies have suggested a link between loneliness and the occurrence of cardiovascular problems, inflammation in the body and memory impairment, which alone has several negative effects. For example, researchers have observed changes in some genes of the human immune system alone. Some of the key genes involved in antiviral reactions and the production of antibodies undergo changes in their bodies that weaken the immune system against viral attacks. In general, due to the increasing prevalence of cancer and the importance of psychological factors such as stress, anxiety, depression, etc. in creating and worsening the condition of these patients, as well as the study and comparison of other influential factors such as loneliness that is associated with some diseases. Such as the occurrence of cardiovascular problems, inflammation in the body, memory impairment, etc. have been identified. This study will also seek to answer the fundamental question of whether there is a difference between perceived stress, anxiety and loneliness in breast cancer patients and normal people?

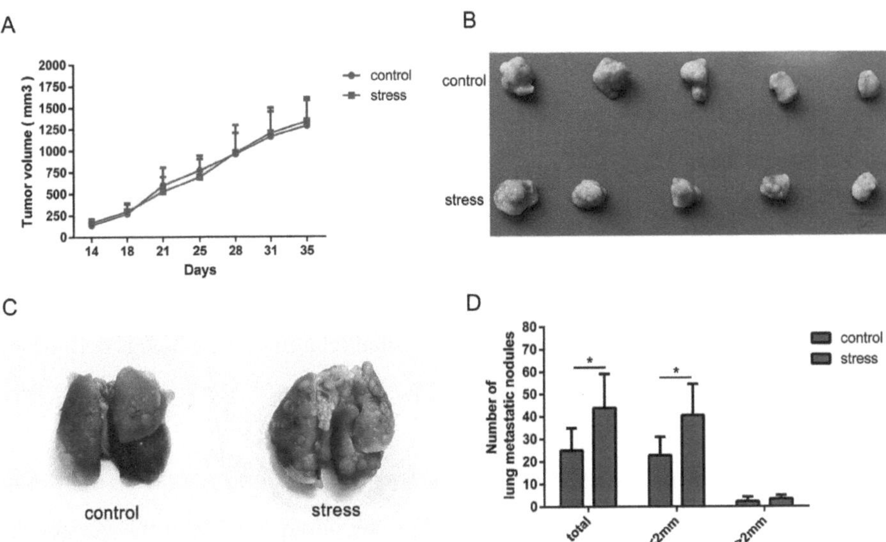

Figure 23. Chronic stress promotes EMT-mediated metastasis through activation of STAT3 signaling pathway

Theoretical and operational definition of variables

✓ **Perceived stress**

Conceptual definition: Anything that the subject perceives as a psychological pressure on his mind or body.

Operational definition: The score that subjects receive from the perceived stress scale. The measurement scale of this variable is distance.

✓ **Worry**

Conceptual definition: Concern is defined as a circle of very negative emotion that is associated with intolerance of thoughts and images and represents an attempt to use mental problem solving as an issue that has an important outcome, but has negative consequences. It is more sensitive.

Operational definition of anxiety: In this study, anxiety refers to the score that subjects receive from 24 items of the anxiety questionnaire. The measurement scale of this variable is distance.

✓ **Alone**

Conceptual definition: In fact, the feeling of loneliness can be considered as a perceived inadequacy and weakness in interpersonal relationships, which is defined as the difference between the desired level and the existing level of social relations, and the greater the difference, the greater the feeling of loneliness.

Operational definition of loneliness: The score that subjects receive from the Adult Socio-Emotional Feeling Scale (SELSA-S). The measurement scale of this variable is distance.

Chapter III

Theoretical foundations and research background

Introduction

For a long time, he was an uninvited guest who caused many people suffering. Because there was no medication, the chances of survival were very low. Infectious diseases, which were common due to poor hygiene, have been a major cause of human mortality for the past few centuries. With the spread of urbanization and the promotion of urban culture, human life gradually took on a different color. People care more about their health than ever before and try to avoid getting sick and pathogens as much as possible, but as people's lifestyles change, the cause of death also changes dramatically due to disease. The cause of death changed from acute infectious diseases to chronic diseases that have a gradual and long-term onset. Chronic diseases such as cancer, diabetes and heart disease, etc. are not caused by a single cause, and several underlying factors are involved in its onset and progression, and prevention of these diseases is not possible without knowing all the causes. We have all heard the horrible and scary word cancer and we know what problems and challenges it is synonymous with for the life of the sufferer and his family. Although many cancers can be controlled today with different methods and treatments that are evolving day by day, but nevertheless, this disease is consuming a large number of people every day. We all have to accept that we are potentially at risk for cancer. It may be hard for most people to believe this. What increases their risk of cancer is their unhealthy behaviors and their own negative mental states. Unhealthy lifestyle, chronic worries, and low self-efficacy are among the psychological variables that predispose people to cancer. Tobacco and alcohol consumption, high-risk sexual behaviors, lack of adequate physical activity, unhealthy and high-fat diet are among the lifestyle factors that researchers and experts believe can lead to disease by interfering with other factors. Long-term worries, lack of self-confidence, and feelings of inability to control the situation, with their impact on immune system function, can certainly increase a person's risk of cancer in the long run.

The history of studies on stress and cancer dates back to BC. Studies conducted before BC show that depressed people are more at risk for breast cancer. In recent decades, the role of stress due to its effect on sex hormones and the body's immune system has been re-examined by researchers. Stress affects the metabolism of estrogen in the body, and a disorder in the metabolism of this hormone can lead to cancers related to the female organs. According to some studies, stress gradually affects the immune system and impairs the body's immune system, and the result can lead to the growth of cancer cells in the body, because the immune system fights against the proliferation of this the cells become weak. Accordingly, stress can be a trigger for cancer. Cancer cells form regularly in the body on a daily basis, but are collected from the body in a certain order. Coping with stress and life problems can disrupt this order. Paying attention to the intensity and form of stress that a person endures and in what rank and position a person is in terms of personality is effective in relation to cancer and its effect. Some researchers believe that severe stress can contribute to cancer, while others believe that long-term and chronic stress may contribute to this type of disease. However, research shows that stress in both forms has an effect on the risk of cancer. It has not been proven that stress increases or decreases the risk of breast cancer. But most studies are moving toward proving increased risk. The idea that cancer may be related to stress is raised around 200 BC, said a scientist named Galen. Melancholic women are more prone to breast cancer. In 1759, a surgeon named Guy emphasized that life-threatening events could lead to cancer. Some studies have not only shown an association between breast cancer and emotional factors as well as stressful life events, but also suggested an increased risk in younger women. This is especially important in our country, where the average age of breast cancer is lower than in Western countries. Other studies, in addition to stressful events, have suggested that the lack of social support during traumatic events is also involved in breast cancer. Ancient Greek physicians have believed in the relationship between mind and body since two thousand years ago. Cancer is one of the diseases that has long been associated with personality. Greek physician Galen observed that melancholic women are more prone to cancer than aggressive women. Jund Ron wrote that cancer appears after deep fear and sorrow. Vega 1759 concluded that women with mental and hysterical problems were more likely to develop cancer, but that cancer-prone naive women were more likely to develop cancer, in addition to having been involved in many catastrophic situations. In

1854, Amosat mentioned the role of Ali Sog Vangrani in the incidence of cancer. In general, until the nineteenth century, cancer was associated with the lack of depression associated with Mullah Nekulia.

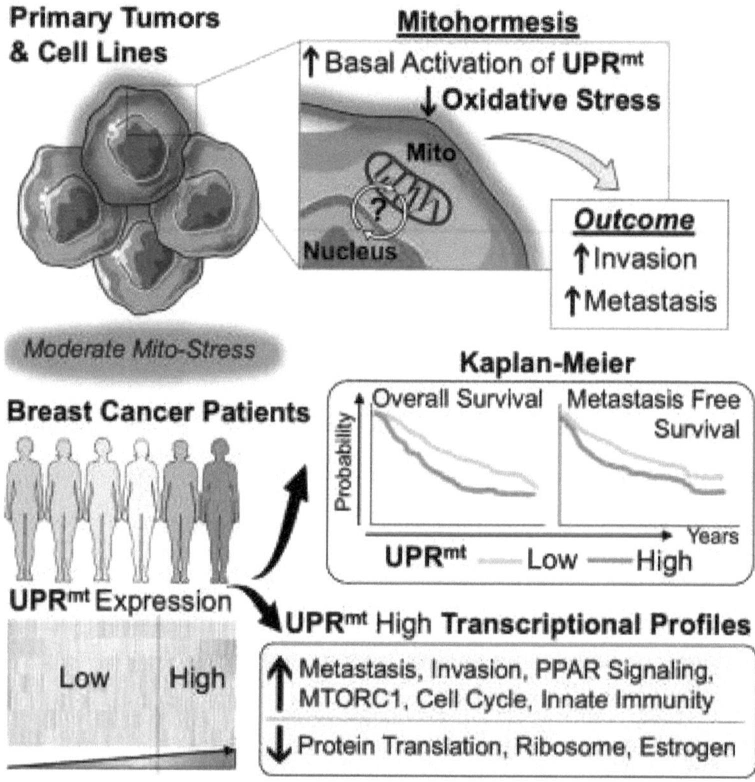

Figure 24. Mitohormesis Primes Tumor Invasion and Metastasis

Early studies in the twentieth century

In the second half of the twentieth century, this field was reactivated. One of the first researchers in this field is Lee Shan and his colleagues. After studying 500 cancer patients, they found that these patients had an important relationship in the past where they could express their feelings of anger and aggression. They have a feeling of self-loathing and high self-esteem. Unresolved problems related to parental death are long gone. Early studies place more emphasis on the masochistic personality structure, stating that people prone to cancer have no way of directly expressing anger or its sublimated form. Bloomberg-Wallis reports that defensive and highly anxious patients show rapid cancer growth through motor outflow. In addition to being defensive, these patients have a calm appearance in times of severe discomfort. The general characteristics of these people in addition to frustration are summarized as follows. Lack of important relationships, inability to express hostility in favor of others, feelings of hopelessness, suppression of emotions. Miller and Jonesh examined the cancer patient and its association with pre-disease emotional stress. Green and Miller cited personal loss as a major precursor to cancer. Others have identified depression as the most common sign of cancer.

This research led to the second half of the twentieth century, known as the period of the emergence of research on cancer personality correlations. The main characteristics mentioned in the research of this course are: excessive cooperation, satisfying the needs of others, lack of courage, avoidance of conflict, emotional inhibition such as anger and anxiety, use of defense mechanisms of repression and denial, self-sacrifice, rigidity and rigidity Being prone to experience depression and hopelessness. It has categorized these features into two main categories. Emotional inhibition such as fear and anger and behaviors commensurate with these emotions, inappropriate coping mechanisms that lead to failure, feelings of hopelessness and helplessness, and ultimately depression and despair.

Modern research approaches

The existence of methodological deficiencies and the emergence of holistic approaches in psychological and theoretical research on hereditary vulnerability/ stress led researchers to control the personality factors involved in cancer susceptible individuals through controlled research and using components of hereditary vulnerability to stress. To study. Eisenhower and Kissen were among the first to study the relationship between personality factors and cancer using controlled methods. Eisenhower believes that stressors are not stressful in themselves, but it is the individual reactions of individuals that determine how stressful events are, and the experience of stress may vary from person to person depending on personality factors. Thus, the stress experienced by the individual is the result of a combination of stressors and inherited morbidity (personality). Eisenhower refers to personality, characteristics (primary factors), types (high level factors) of attitudes, defense mechanisms and other non-cognitive aspects of behavior and its biological and environmental underlying factors. According to this view, recognizing and distinguishing the contribution of hereditary morbidity and morbidity / stress is very important. It is assumed that most of the components of inherited vulnerability are some aspects of negative excitability (such as neuroticism or anxiety and depression) that interacts with stress/disaster and produces the ultimate morbid or psychological effects. Based on theories of vulnerability, it is believed that there are a number of general personality factors that act in the opposite direction of disease to health.

These factors are called H or (Health). There are factors that work against cancer and coronary heart disease, which are called D or differences because of their differences. One of these concepts is alexithymia, which, despite the difficulty in identifying and describing emotions and distinguishing bodily emotions, is characterized by limited lattice processes and is positively associated with neuroticism, negatively with extraversion, and positively associated with physical complaints.

Self-regulation (self-regulation) is another concept. Low sympathetic arousal in response to cyclical pressures is another health variable. Courage and perseverance are also positive signs of predicting health. Optimism, struggle and self-efficacy are also among these concepts. The concept of dependent personality is also a complex feature of health. Bolger and Schilling showed that coping and responsiveness to stressors accounted for more than 40% of the difference in discomfort between subjects with high and low neuroticism. Kessler et al. Believe that in addition to them, there may be other personality variables that can act indirectly through these factors and as social support that reduce stress, but in fact a function of variables such as Extraversion, neuroticism, the center of control, and so on. A new era of research began with the work of Kissen and Eisenhower. They followed the experimental method. In their study, they studied the relationship between lung cancer and emotional inhibition. People at risk for cancer scored low on the Madzley questionnaire, indicating their emotional inhibition.

Keyson and Raw repeated this study several times and obtained similar results. These people are six times more likely to develop lung cancer than those who scored high on the neuroticism scale. Caeson says the lack of an outlet for emotional outbursts leads to lung cancer, even with the slightest exposure to smoking. Eisenhower believes that low scores on neurosis may be due to two reasons.

A person with a low score is really stable and experiences little anxiety and depression. The person experiences and denies them while experiencing high anxiety and depression. Therefore, the actual and net inhibition results are expected to be higher than this. Experimental studies of emotional inhibition support the second hypothesis. The second characteristic is the tendency to fail in the face of stress or surrender and the feeling of hopelessness and helplessness. Schmal and Iker examined women with suspected cervical cells before the diagnosis and found with a 79% accuracy the risk of developing cervical cancer in people with a high potential for frustration or frustration six months before the spots formed. Suspicious predicted.

Types of cancers are a wide range of diseases, each of which has its own etiology, treatment plan and prognosis. Most people with cancer experience a period of stress. In some patients, this stress resolves spontaneously and does not lead to long-term mental problems and can be considered as a normal adjustment reaction, but some patients experience more severe mental problems that It reduces their quality of life and daily performance. These psychologically severe mental problems usually occur as part of an adaptive disorder, major depressive disorder, or an anxiety disorder. Cancer treatment is also associated with a number of psychological pressures, some of which reduce the quality of life and lead to anxiety or depression. For example, patients often rate the psychological side effects of treatment such as anger, anxiety, or worry more severely than physical side effects such as hair loss and nausea. Some patients even give up chemotherapy. Cancer crises cause imbalances in the mind, body and soul, but the most common during this period is a feeling of despair and hopelessness for the patient. Among these, breast cancer is the most common, deadly and emotionally and psychologically most effective cancer among women. Breast cancer is an abnormal growth of cells in which the cells grow out of control and overgrow normally, forming tumors called tumors. These lumps are often painless and stiff in the upper part. And external breasts begin.

In 2002, about one million and one hundred and fifty thousand new cases of breast cancer were reported worldwide, and about 1.5 million new cases are predicted to begin in 2010. According to a national report of 7 Iranian cancer cases registered during the last 4 decades, the increase in the incidence of breast cancer has made it one of the most malignant among Iranian women and affects Iranian women a decade earlier than their counterparts in developed countries.

The incidence of this cancer is increasing rapidly in women 50 years of age and older. From January 1998 to December 2005, the incidence of cancer in Iranian women was one year, and Iranians were 22 per 100,000 women, ranging in age from 40 to 49 years. The nature of this disease is such that it endangers the identity and female personality of the patients and causes them with issues such as anxiety, depression, despair, feeling of social isolation, fear of the reaction of the spouse if married, worry about marriage if single, fear from sterilization to death and apprehension and .... Makes face.

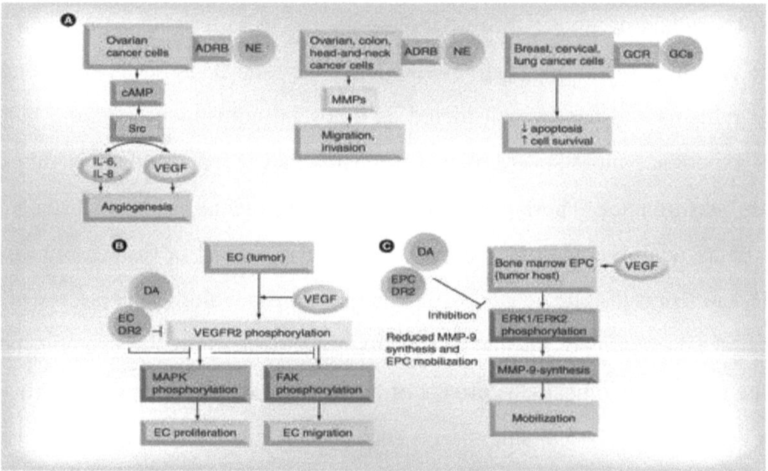

Figure 25. Impact of stress on cancer metastasis

Epidemiology

Breast cancer is an important epidemiological issue with global spread. Women in industrialized countries have a higher risk of infection than others, with Japan being an exception. Diagnosing breast cancer is one of the most pleasurable events that can happen in a woman's life. But instead of letting disease and stress overwhelm you, try to control it yourself. According to doctors, the fear of breast cancer is a natural and widespread reaction, part of which is due to the increase in public awareness about this disease. In addition to the physical dimension, these patients also suffer from the psychological effects of breast cancer.

Reasons

In this disease, malignant proliferation of virtual epithelial cells or mammary lobules occurs. Like all epithelial malignancies, the incidence of cancer increases almost with age, but the slope of this curve decreases with the age of menopause. The age of onset of menstruation, the first pregnancy and also menopause are three important dates influencing the incidence of breast cancer in women. Thus, the younger the age of onset of menstruation, the older the age of the first pregnancy, and the older the age of onset of menopause, the higher the risk, which indicates that the cancer is dependent on sex hormones. Women who started menstruating at the age of 16 About 50-60% of people who menstruate at the age of 12 develop breast cancer. Similarly, this risk reaches 35% in women whose menopause is 10 years earlier than their normal average age (52) or in women who have had an early period due to ovarian resection. The risk of breast cancer is one-third of cases in which normal menopause occurs at age 50 or older. Also, people who have experienced their first pregnancy under the age of 20 have a 30-40% lower risk of cancer than women in Noli Par. This is due to the constant exposure to internal estrogen in the absence of a sufficient concentration of progesterone. Therefore, the length of the menstrual period, and especially that part of the period that occurs before the first pregnancy, are effective factors in causing breast cancer. This factor can be responsible for 70-80% of the reasons for the difference in the incidence of breast cancer between different nationalities. For example, patients with breast cancer in Iran have different patterns than patients in Western countries. The average age of these patients in our country is lower than others. According to several studies, the presence of a family history of breast cancer and marital loss were two important factors influencing Iranian patients. The majority of young patients in Iran can be largely justified by the young population structure of our country. The two factors of menstruation in older age and the first pregnancy in younger age are important protective factors against infection in older age.

Therefore, in the presence of these two factors, the prevalence of this cancer tends to younger ages. In the meantime, especially during the first full-term pregnancy, it is the most important protective factor. According to research results, not giving birth reduces the risk of breast cancer at a younger age and, conversely, increases its risk at an older age. Geographical studies on the incidence and mortality of breast cancer have shown that the risk factors for this disease are different in different areas, and for breast cancer, mainly environmental factors are stronger than genetic factors.

Hereditary factors

The role of hereditary and genetic factors as predisposing factors in breast cancer has been confirmed. One-third of all patients have a positive history of breast cancer in one or more of their first- or second-degree dependents. People who have a sister or mother with breast cancer have a 4 times higher risk. But this does not mean that if your mother or first-degree relatives have a history of infection, you will definitely get it too. Breast cancer caused by genes involved in the disease and hereditary factors is commonly seen in several relatives under the age of 40 and in one or both breasts. The different genes identified can determine the histological characteristics and severity of tumor invasion.

Diet

Consumption of high-fat and fried foods doubles the risk of breast cancer. The quality and quantity of dietary fat both affect the development of this disease. It has also been linked to moderate alcohol consumption and the incidence of this disease, the mechanism of which is still unknown.

Hormone consumption

Determining the potential role of hormones in breast cancer is important, as millions of women are regularly taking oral contraceptives or taking hormone replacement therapy during menopause. It is believed that taking oral contraceptive pills, even for a long time, has no effect on increasing the incidence of breast cancer. But studies also show that long-term use of combination pills in people who are very young or have not been pregnant can be effective in causing this cancer.

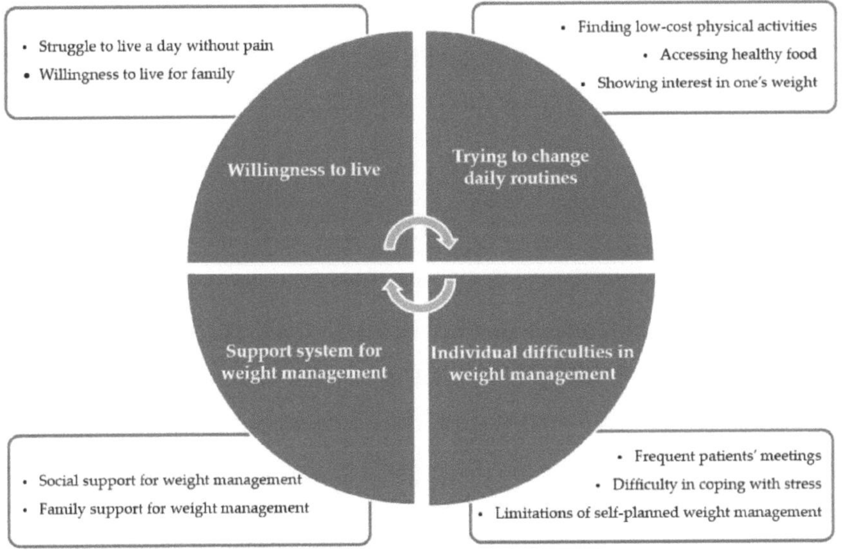

Figure 26. Photovoice-Based Assessment of Weight Management Experiences

However, they suggest that the role of these factors in causing cancer, even if positive, is very small (in contrast, oral contraceptives play a protective role against ovarian epithelial tumors and endometrial cancer). Studies by the World Health Organization show that the use of injectable contraceptives has no effect on increasing the risk of breast cancer. It is not yet known whether hormone replacement therapy (HRT) changes the risk of breast cancer if there is a family history of breast cancer or positive cells in a previous biopsy. Some researchers have found that pre- and post-menopausal estrogen use is associated with a slight increase in the risk of breast cancer. Especially if there is a history of benign breast disease, but if you take estrogen with progesterone, there is not enough information about the amount of this effect. By and large, high weight is associated with breast cancer. The risk in obese women is 2-5.1 times higher than others, which is related to menopause.

History of primary cancer

In women who have a previous positive sign of breast cancer, the risk of developing the opposite breast is 3-4 times higher. Also, despite a previous history of ovarian or uterine carcinoma, the risk of breast cancer increases 3.1-4.1 times.

Radiation

Young women who have been exposed to radiation to the chest (for multiple fluoroscopic or therapeutic purposes) have a higher risk of developing the disease. But at the age of over 30, this amount reaches its lowest level. The risk of multiple low-dose irradiations is the same as for a single high-dose irradiation. Less than 1% of breast cancers are caused by radiological diagnostic procedures. Radiology to treat breast cancer may also increase the risk of involvement. Following radiation to treat cervical cancer reduces the risk of breast cancer. This is because of the decrease in estrogen levels.

Factors influencing the course of the disease

The most important factors are the ones that determine the staging of patients. Other variables include estrogen and progesterone receptors. Receptor-deficient tumors are more prone to recurrence. Tumor growth criteria, tumor classification histologically, molecular changes in the tumor, and proteins involved in invasion are other influential factors. There is disagreement about the choice of combination therapies, including chemotherapy and hormone therapy. Different treatment regimens are prescribed for different groups of patients. For example, a woman who is menopausal and is positive for lymph node involvement and the presence of hormone receptors, regardless of other tumors, is advised to administer tamoxifen (anti-estrogen) without chemotherapy. Tamoxifen is very effective in preventing the recurrence of estrogen receptor-type breast cancers.

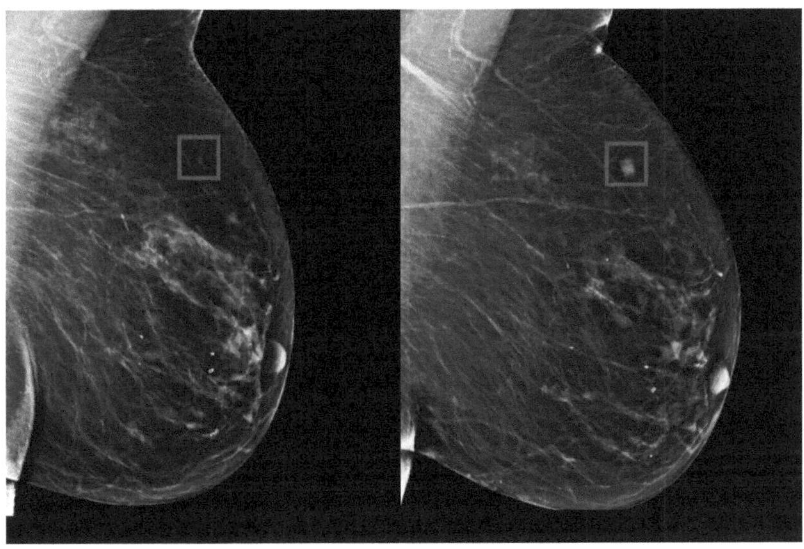

Figure 27. Using AI to predict breast cancer and personalize care

Breast cancer is a serious and deadly disease that can lead to death if not treated properly. Australian women die of breast cancer more than any other cancer, and one in nine Canadian women will develop breast cancer in their lifetime. In Scotland, breast cancer is the second most common cause of death in women.

Types of Cancer

- ✓ **Invasive:** The basement membrane limiting the tumor is torn.
- ✓ **Noninvasive:** The basement membrane limiting the tumor is not torn.

Breast cancer classification

Non-invasive cancers themselves fall into two categories:

- ✓ Ductal carcinoma in situ (DCIS)
- ✓ Lobular Carcinoma in situ (LCIS)

Invasive cancer itself is divided into six categories:

- ✓ Invasive ductal carcinoma
- ✓ Invasive lobular carcinoma
- ✓ Medullary lobular carcinoma
- ✓ Colloid lobular carcinoma
- ✓ Tobular lobular carcinoma
- ✓ Other type

Staging of breast cancer

There are several factors that determine the most appropriate treatment for you. These factors include clinical history, age, general health status, and the type and extent of cancer. The rate of cancer spread is known as the cancer stage.

Different stages of breast cancer

Stage 1: The tumor is 2 cm or less in diameter and does not extend beyond the breast.

Stage 2: The tumor is 2 to 5 cm in diameter and may have spread to the axillary lymph nodes.

Stage 3: The tumor is larger than 5 cm and has spread to the axillary lymph nodes more than stage 2 and may have spread to other lymph nodes or tissues near the breast.

Stage 4: The cancer has spread (metastasized) to other parts of the body. These organs are often the lungs, bones, liver or brain.

Therapeutic methods

The four most common types of breast cancer treatment are surgery, radiation therapy, chemotherapy, and hormone therapy. The type of treatment largely depends on the patient's health status and stage of the disease. Surgery is the most common treatment for breast cancer and different surgical methods can be used. The types of these surgeries, from the most detailed to the most extensive, are listed in the section on types of breast cancer surgeries.

What is stress?

Stress can be considered as psychological, physical, emotional, behavioral reactions of a person to any perceived internal or environmental threat or pressure. He has defined stress as follows: It is the body's vague response to any pressure that affects it, whether it produces pleasure or pain. Saliyeh pointed out that whether a good situation is imagined, such as a job promotion, or a bad situation, such as unemployment, the physiological response to this arousal is very similar. According to Saliyeh, the body cannot distinguish between good and bad stress. In a single situation, two people may have completely different perceptions. The perception of a stressful situation is the same. Stress is closely related to the leading cause of death, including heart disease, headache, accident, liver cirrhosis, suicide, and laryngeal problems. Stress is part of every human being's natural problem. We actually face three types of stress. Ustress, nostril, distress. Ustress is the same as good stress and occurs in a situation that one finds motivating or inspiring. Users give us the energy and motivation to fulfill our responsibilities and achieve our goals.

Education, marriage to the person we love, career advancement and career change are among these. Nostress refers to a sensory stimulus that has no effect on the brain. Stress that is neither good nor bad, like hearing the news of an earthquake in a remote part of the world, can fall into this category. Distress is a state of anxiety. This type of stress is bad and is often used as stress. Distress is a constant experience of drowning in responsibilities. Distortion of movement in the tunnel is a problem without the end of the tunnel being known. Financial problems, conflict in interpersonal relationships, over-commitment, managing a chronic illness or experiencing a trauma.

Stress symptoms can be divided into four dimensions

1. Physical or physiological dimensions such as palpitations, shortness of breath, hot, cold, dry mouth and throat, paleness, nausea, vomiting, recurrence of urination, hand tremors, cold palms and soles, muscle contraction and stiffness, fatigue Excessive, anorexia, digestive problems, variable or chronic pain, lack of energy, sleep disturbance.

2. Psychological dimensions such as anxiety, depression, impatience, anger, sensitivity, decreased tolerance threshold, lack of vitality and vitality, decreased concentration, memory impairment, dissatisfaction with self and environment and others, aggression, pessimism, feeling of failure, feeling helpless, feeling hopeless.

3. Social dimension such as reduction of social relations, incompatibility in social relations, loss of social status, loss of avoidance of social situations, abandonment of group recreational activities, non-participation in meetings and parties.

4. Spiritual dimension such as reduction of spiritual interests, conflict with one's existence, conflict with the meaning of life, reduction of creative activities, conflict with human beliefs.

Factors that can produce stress include:

1. Environmental factors such as noise, bad weather or natural resources, traffic, pollution.

2. Social factors such as financial problems, interpersonal disputes, loss of a loved one.

3. Physiological factors such as puberty, physical changes during adolescence, illness, accident, sleep disorders, smoking and addictive substances.

4. Individual factors such as our perception of events, decision making, negative attitude, perfectionism, competition, self-criticism.

5. Coping with stress is both emotion-oriented and problem-oriented. Women use the emotion-oriented method more and men use the problem-oriented method more.

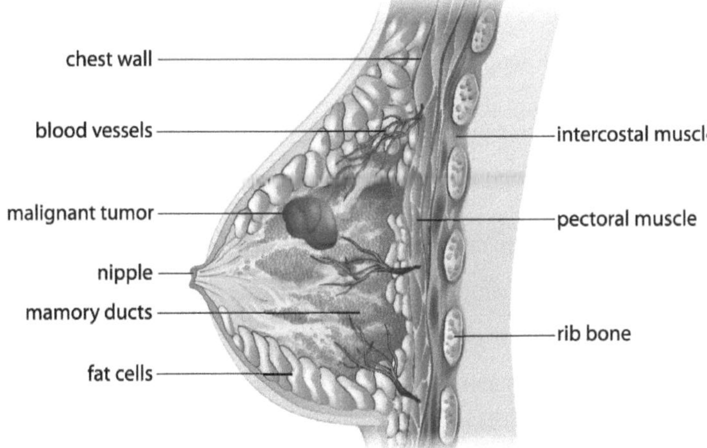

Figure 28. Breast Cancer • types, diagnosis, treatments

1- Emotion-oriented: These are confrontations that aim to calm yourself down and achieve calmness. Religious prayers and confrontations, giving a new and positive meaning to stress, heartache with those around and close, limited expression of emotions, distraction, inner conversation, engaging in mental activities, engaging in physical activities.

2- Problem-oriented: Efforts and activities to eliminate or minimize stress, use problem-solving skills, think about stress, plan, eliminate unnecessary activities and focus on stress and existing problems to maximize Concentrate, be patient instead of using hasty and impulsive solutions, guide and consult others, seek information.

A group of people also deal with their stress inconsistently, which include: resorting to drugs, performing impulsive behaviors without thinking and contemplation, giving up activities and giving up trying (hopelessness), and wishing thinking.

Albert Ellis believed that stress-related behaviors are due to perception and can be changed. Ellis believed that all stimuli sent to the brain undergo a process of change and interpretation. When the stimulus is interpreted sufficiently threateningly, it produces a negative thought, in which case logic loses its meaning.

As a result, a destructive attitude against oneself is reinforced. Ellis believed that people could be trained to change stress-related perceptions (irrational thoughts) into positive attitudes, which would reduce the severity of stress. This is called cognitive reconstruction. According to research and studies conducted on people, it was concluded that positive thoughts cause people to accept situations better and experience less stress, and to cope with the resulting stress and overcome their stress. Psychologists use the term complementary prediction to describe the relationship between their beliefs, perceptions, and related behaviors. They believe that if we predict a situation satisfactorily and well, it will be to our advantage and we will pass that situation without stress and we will succeed, and if we predict a bad situation and have a negative belief in it, and it is the result of self-disappointment that prepares the scene for a stressful situation, and the result is inevitably negative.

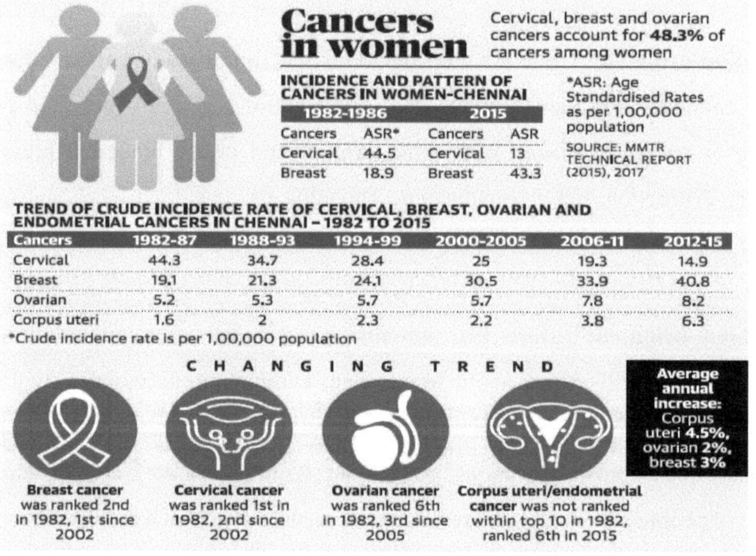

	1982-1986		2015	
Cancers	ASR*	Cancers	ASR	
Cervical	44.5	Cervical	13	
Breast	18.9	Breast	43.3	

TREND OF CRUDE INCIDENCE RATE OF CERVICAL, BREAST, OVARIAN AND ENDOMETRIAL CANCERS IN CHENNAI – 1982 TO 2015

Cancers	1982-87	1988-93	1994-99	2000-2005	2006-11	2012-15
Cervical	44.3	34.7	28.4	25	19.3	14.9
Breast	19.1	21.3	24.1	30.5	33.9	40.8
Ovarian	5.2	5.3	5.7	5.7	7.8	8.2
Corpus uteri	1.6	2	2.3	2.2	3.8	6.3

*Crude incidence rate is per 1,00,000 population

Figure 29. Stress Increases Risk of Breast, Cervical and Ovarian Cancer

Stress

Definition of stress

Stress refers to a quality of experience created by personal-environment interaction through pre-arousal or under-arousal and is limited to psychological or physiological helplessness.

Mason has identified three definitions of stress:

1- The internal state of the organism (which sometimes refers to the pressure of pain).

2- An external event (stressor).

3- An experience called the interaction of person and environment.

In other words, some people consider stress as a response to environmental conditions, which is defined based on various criteria such as emotional distress, difficulty in functioning or physiological changes such as increased skin conduction or increased levels of certain hormones. In the first case, physiological and emotional changes occur in the person. Physiological reactions involve the central nervous system, peripherals, the immune system, and the endocrine system. Stress stimulates the body's sympathetic system, thus preparing the body for activity. Blood flows from the internal organs to the brain. Increased heart rate, blood pressure and respiration cause more oxygen to reach the brain and muscles, and high blood sugar increases energy, all of which lead to more mental and physical activity.

This stimulation of the sympathetic nervous system is called the fight-or-flight response. It is believed that this reaction is a general response to any kind of stress (physical or social) and the body responds to all kinds of threats in the same way, while at that moment the reaction may be irrelevant. Kenen also hypothesized for the first time that the perception of a threat activates the thalamus, which in turn activates the pituitary gland, which secretes the hormones adrenaline and noradrenaline from the adrenal gland. By eliminating the threat, the activity of the second state of stress event is related to the external environment. Early research was on natural disasters and war, and later on important life events, such as marriage, divorce, burnout, or starting a new job, expanded on stressors.

Finally, stress is an experience that results from the interaction between the individual in the environment, especially interactions in which there is a mismatch between individual resources and the perceived challenge or need. In this case, in order for physiological or emotional reactions to occur, the person must be aware of the stress factor (threat, lack, challenge) and this knowledge must be aroused. Stress can threaten a person's well-being and survival, and can lead to physical or mental illness or adaptation. According to Monat research, why a person reacts negatively to a stress depends on many factors, including the individual's response to the stressor. The perception of stress depends on the extent of the pressures and the number of resources that people have to deal with them, and Wolfulk Richardson stated that stress is a cognitive experience that is related to a person's perception of their relationship with the environment.

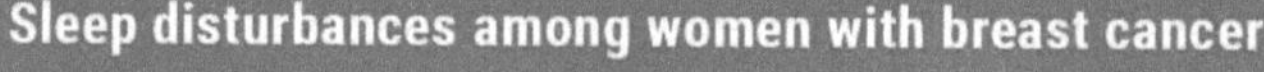

Figure 30. Tailored interventions may mitigate sleep disturbances among women with breast cancer

Theoretical issues raised regarding the stress process

Several theories about the stress process have been proposed, which we will discuss briefly.

Lachman proposed an autonomous and behavioral learning theory to explain the stress process. Lachmann argues that the primary source of frequency and intensity of psychological responses to stress is a response to the fact that over time the slightest amount of stress causes inappropriate responses to the stressors (if one learns to overreact to stress, this Increased response will be enhanced whenever stress occurs.

Schwartzick proposed a system model for stress, stating that whenever communication between specific parts of a system is disturbed, that system is disrupted.

This model is based on four stages

1- The pressures that the environment puts on the person.

2- Regulatory functions of the brain.

3- Activation of special bodily systems according to the nature of environmental pressures.

4- If this process continues, negative physical loops about the balance mechanism will enter the game and put pressure on the brain to perform its management.

Kaplan states that a person's response to stress is understood in three stages:

Step 1: Behavior that changes a stressful environment and enables a person to escape from that environment.

The second step is to learn behavior in order to acquire new capacities to change external conditions and their consequences.

Stage 3: Behavior within the psyche that the organism inevitably copes with the event and its consequences.

Lazarus stated that a person's perception plays an important role in what he calls mental stressful events. According to Lazarus, stress is an interaction between the person and the environment and the person's assessment of threatening or challenging events. Lazarus suggested that stress reactions can be classified into four main types: impaired emotion, behavioral motor reactions, changes in cognitive function, and physiological changes. According to Lazarus, stress is related to excitement and the adaptation of one's experience to stress, and stress responses depend on learning, growth, and culture. This view suggests that stress will occur when both the challenging situation puts pressure on Angizia to evaluate and there are not enough resources to deal with the situation. Increase and develop. The first group is tangible resources such as houses and cars, which are in line with physical needs and improve the situation. The second group sources resources such as marital status and job security. The third group are sources of personal characteristics. Many personal characteristics are associated with stress resistance and psychological and physical well-being. These resources include positive self-esteem, a sense of inner control, optimism, efficiency, self-efficacy, mastery, and quality of attachment. The fourth group is called energy sources, which include money, time, knowledge and awareness. There are several approaches to stress based on cognitive theory. Ellis states that irrational beliefs lead to stress. Beck argued that stress is an interpretation of events, and that Mitchenbaum also believed that internal conversations and self-thinking lead to the experience of people experiencing stress.

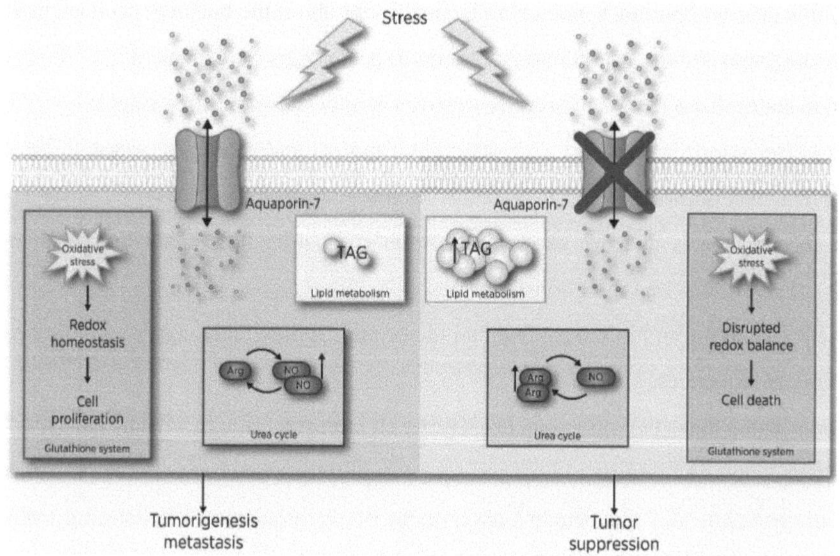

Figure 31. Regulates the Response to Cellular Stress in Breast Cancer

General models of stress

Despite many definitions of stress, there are three general theories or models. These models are called stimulus-oriented, response-oriented, and exchangeable.

1- Stimulus model: Stimulus theorists think that environmental factors cause stress. Environmental stressors are defined as those that lead to psychological helplessness, behavioral damage, or the breakdown of a person's performance and poor perception. Stimulus modeling research is based on the idea that major events cause change and that these changes lead to a range of physical ailments. In this model, more attention is paid to the specific characteristics of a stressors and it is stated that each critical event has its own unique stressors that may be physical, social, role or task. So that the coping resources bother the person and trigger a specific stress response. The stimulus model has been criticized for abandoning the idea that non-major events may also contribute to stress.

2- Responsive model: The responsive model was proposed by Hans Selie and became known as (general syndrome of compromise). Selieh believed that stress is a defensive response and goes through three stages. Warning, resistance and wear. In the alert phase, the body defends itself against annoying conditions by activating the sympathetic nervous system. The alert response moves the body to respond in battle or flight and is used as a short-term adaptive response in emergency situations. When the resistance stage arrives, the body gets used to the strassor and prepares itself for defense. At this stage, although the person does not state that he is under stress, but the organism does not function well and eventually becomes ill. In the exhaustion stage, the physical resource is depleted and the organism is unable to maintain a level of readiness. Clay was distinguished between stressor (stimulus) and stress (response). Selia did not pay attention to the nature of the stressor and paid more attention to the physiological response and growth of the disease. In this model, Selia did not agree with the role of emotions and cognition and focused only on physiological reactions. Sally believed that all organisms, regardless of how the situation appears, show a non-specific response to annoying stimuli. Modern psychological theories, on the other hand, consider a person's interpretation of situations to be a major determinant of stressors.

Exchange model

In the stress exchange model, stress theorists consider the product of the individual's relationship with the environment. Traditional theories consider stress as a process based on perceived pressures on a person and their capacity for response. This model is different from stimulus and response-oriented models. Because it has to do with a person's perception.

Lazarus and Folkman proposed a model of coping with five major components:

- ✓ Individual and effective environmental factors
- ✓ Cognitive assessments
- ✓ Stress
- ✓ Coping responses
- ✓ Short-term and long-term adaptive results.

In the exchange model, stress is the result of a perceived imbalance between pressures and demands and resources and can range from everyday parts to major life events.

Causes of stress: life changes and troubles

Stress is present in all areas of life and everywhere to varying degrees. The main causes of stress are:

1- Life changes: Important life-changing events, such as marriage, the death of a family member, or relocation, can be stressful, according to Holmes. A short time can have adverse consequences for mental health. All life changes, including marriage, the death of a family member, changes in daily working hours, and even changes in the hours of movement of vehicles are stressful, and if the level of stress exceeds the body's ability to adapt, it can endanger his mental health and even Lead to physical illness. Holmes and Rahe have developed a scale that includes 41 stressful situations in order of importance and can predict the relationship between life changes and mental health. The authors value each situation numerically, thereby creating a scale that evaluates life changes. People with scores higher than 300 on this scale are more likely to be mentally depressed than those with moderate scores, as well as those with cardiovascular disease and so on. The authors believe that an increase in the sum of the total scores can be a prognosis for an increase in unfortunate life events.

2- Failure: Failure is the hypothetical state of a person who has encountered an obstacle in the pursuit of one of his natural goals. Even if someone feels cheated, they will still fail. The reason that failure is considered hypothetical is that gravity cannot be studied directly. Its failure and severity of weakness cannot be inferred from behavior. According to the school of psychoanalysis, failure is the state of a person who, for internal or external reasons, is deprived of libido (the substance or motor force of life instincts). Thus, in psychoanalysis, failure results from deprivation of physiological drivers or motives. When we say that failure may have internal or external causes, we mean that the obstacle can be in the person or outside of him. For example, a man or a woman is not allowed to work in some jobs or to be present in some places. The university faces an internal obstacle. Short stature can also be an internal barrier to entering military careers. Failure, if severe and lasting, is likely to endanger a person's mental health and lead to physical and mental disorders. But it should not be overlooked that failure is determined by the obstacle in the way of the goal, for example, a worker who has been deprived of sleep for 12 hours or a student who has not been able to attend a meeting due to heavy traffic or road breakdown. Attend the exam, how failed it is. There is no tool to measure people's failure. A certain situation may be suitable for one person who fails and for another person. As some patients do not like to recover, because they know they have to take responsibility.

3- Long-term stress: Stressful situations do not appear only in the form of short-term events such as death or birth. Magnificent or lowly marriages, poor working conditions, or a depressing political climate can also be long-term stressors. However, whether these factors are short-term or long-term, each person reacts differently to them. For example, a worker can work for many years under the domination of an unscrupulous employer, but another worker cannot endure even a month. Everyone's reaction to long-term stressors depends on their assessment of the situation. Personally, divorce, job loss, alcoholism, and financial problems can be stressful for all family members. Social life can also be stressful. Because to find and keep a few friends, we often need a lot of effort and energy. This is especially true for those who are shy or uncomfortable with strangers. Maintaining long-term friendships can also be difficult at times, as long distances, administrative or employment obligations, and marriage limit leisure time and make travel difficult. All of these factors lead to long-term stress. In long-term stress research, most stressors in the workplace or in relation to work have been studied. People are usually stressed out or unable to cope with their co-workers. Therefore, in a society where there are no job security and people are always worried about losing their job or cannot change their place of work and be with people with whom they are comfortable, mental health disappears and goes nowhere. Stress can greatly affect a person and their family members. According to research, a father who is stressed at work is more willing to fight with his family, especially with his son. The effect of this conflict goes so far that the boy also fails in a satisfying relationship with his friends.

4- Life problems: In addition to different types of long-term stress, there are also daily stresses that are attributed to daily work problems. These troubles seem seemingly insignificant and insignificant. Like finding a parking space for cars, standing in line for bread and buses, paying for water, electricity and telephone on time, controlling the number of calls to the city, controlling water and electricity consumption, etc. can become important sources of stress and mental health. Face harmful fluctuations.

5- conflicts: We have said that man fails when he encounters an obstacle in the way of meeting one of his rational needs. If the failure is long-term, one's mental health will be endangered. Therefore, one must somehow overcome one's failure. To overcome failure, either the obstacle must be removed or the goal must be changed. For example, a person who cannot have children either has to seek treatment or resort to selective reproductive methods, or in general, get rid of the idea of having children and seek to establish a kindergarten or have an adopted child. When a person cannot easily decide to do at least one of the two things, he gets a situation called conflict. Conflict, then, is a negative emotional state that arises from the inability to choose at least one of two incompatible goals. In other words, conflict occurs when one cannot choose one of at least two uncompromising ways. Psychologists point to three main types of conflict, each of which brings with it varying degrees of failure. These conflicts are: absorber-absorber, repellent-repellent, absorber-repellent.

Some experts believe that daily troubles are much more stressful than life events. In fact, it can be said that an important event in life happens and daily troubles increase spontaneously. As a result, the event itself becomes more stressful. For example, when marriage or the death of a loved one, the troubles of life increase and the stressful power of marriage or death increases. For this reason, in the Life Transformation Evaluation Scale, 12 points have been given to change of residence and 73 points to divorce. Relocation causes a lot of problems every day, but divorce can cause dozens of problems in the long run. Including being forced to move or leave home by a spouse. It may even be a lot more stressful than the basics of moving or selling a home. All of these important events, and with them all the troubles of life, can be detrimental to mental health, but as mentioned, there are also significant individual differences.

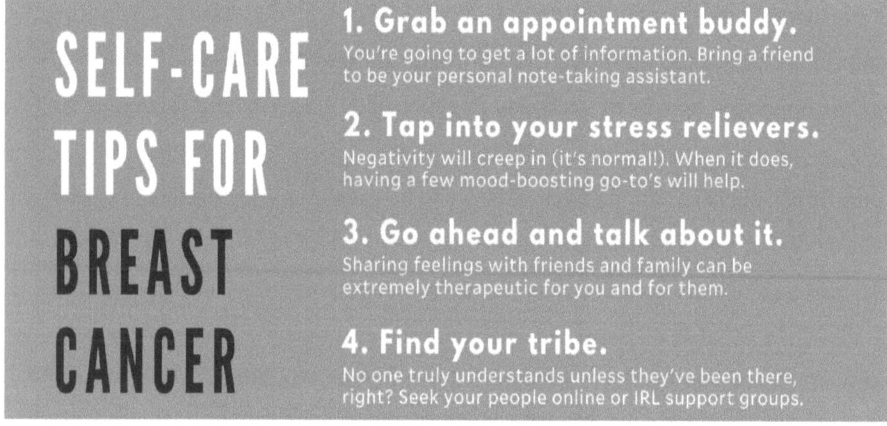

Figure 32. Meditation for Breast Cancer Patients

Types of stress

Stress is divided into three parts. (Physiological, pathological and psychological stresses)

1- Physiological stresses: such as insomnia or excessive fatigue due to overwork or not eating for a long time or working in an unsuitable environment, extreme cold and heat, and doing physical work beyond one's strength and capacity.

2-Pathological stress: such as nervous fatigue, surgery, childbirth, internal infections, sudden change of environment (for the elderly) injuries and injuries and physical illnesses, disorders of the central nervous system such as brain tumors, sudden disorders of the endocrine system Menopause during puberty or menstruation.

3- Psychological stresses: such as intense and sudden emotional states, long worries, lack of coordination in married life, living in an inappropriate environment full of conflict, economic poverty, responsible jobs, cultural pressures.

Components of stress

1- **Biological components of stress:** The body has its own way of dealing with stress. Every threat or challenge that a person perceives in the environment triggers a chain of endocrine events. These events can be conceptualized as two separate responses, one being the sympathetic / adrenal responses with catecholamine secretion and the other pituitary / adrenal responses with corticosteroid secretion. The sympathetic / adrenal response by the sympathetic nervous system sends a message from the brain to the adrenal gland to secrete epinephrine and norepinephrine. This process is the basis of the war and escape response, where the heart rate increases and blood pressure rises. In response, the pituitary / adrenal stimulates the hypothalamus to produce corticotropin-releasing factor (CRE), which is delivered to the pituitary gland through the bloodstream, where the pituitary gland releases corticotropic hormone into the adrenal cortex. Gives up. The adrenal cortex will then secrete the hormone cortisol, but prolonged secretion of this hormone can cause health problems.

2. **Learned components of stress:** The nature of the stress response and how the animal or human responds to stress can be reduced through learning. The ability to predict when a stressful stimulus will occur allows people to relax in the absence of a stressful stimulus. Short rest seems to control the effects of stress. In addition, learning to cope with stress seems to reduce some of the negative effects of stress, such as gastrointestinal ulcers. Evidence suggests that under stress, self-employed and accustomed responses are weakened. Wrong decisions in stressful situations are a good example of how stress can disrupt performance by disrupting attention. Social interactions, especially social conflicts, can be an important source of stress. Studies on organizations in which there is conflict are more. One of the characteristics of such organizations is the lack of common goals as well as the inflexible structure that does not tolerate dissent. Among the characteristics of organizations in which there is no conflict, tolerance of different theories, common goals, and lack of competition can be mentioned. People who work in such organizations are healthier.

3- Cognitive components of stress: According to Lazarus' theory, the initial assessment includes the classification of a stressful event and whether it causes harm, loss, threat or challenge. Secondary evaluation includes evaluation of adaptive resources and available choices. Adaptive strategies are generally either problem-oriented or emotion-oriented. According to Lazarus' theory, whether a person tends to use problem-based or emotion-driven adaptation depends on two other factors. Is the potential threat controllable or not, and if so, does the individual think he or she has the skills to deal with it?

Stress prevention methods

Hassan Selieh, the father of stress research, asks a question at the end of his famous book (The Pressure of Life). He says whether human beings are able to scientifically study the phenomenon of stress to design a detailed program to regulate their behavior to the extent that it can prevent the pressures of life? Or at least reduce its severity? By designing this program, can we smooth out the stress of conflict and effortless effort and have a satisfying and meaningful life? Selieh also answers the question that each person should solve their problems according to their specific personality and environmental characteristics, but in principle, achieving general rules that clarify how stress affects the psyche, each person forward. Equips or relieves stress. Thus, Sally strongly divides the rules and criteria necessary for healthy behavior and the prevention of stress.

1- Short-term goals

Short-term goals are to satisfy desires immediately. Many of these goals are easily achievable and do not require complex planning and long-term learning. These are activities that do not require much effort. Such as enjoying nature through the senses, having fun, walking, walking, various fun games, creative activities such as painting, breathing in the open air, enjoying seeing others or observing their happiness. In these activities, work and rewards are done almost at the same time. It is obvious that these kinds of simple, natural and easy-to-reach pleasures can lead to feelings of happiness and well-being. But the psyche is able to achieve more lasting and deeper satisfaction. In addition, not everyone is able to enjoy natural and simple pleasures such as enjoying nature or music or painting. Therefore, each person should be in search of what is acceptable to his nature and adapts to the construction of his personality. Microscopically observed cells. The most important thing in this kind of pleasures is that they are pure and that they have no specific purpose other than to create happiness and joy in the person. They are not done for profit or profit or for a specific material purpose. All people who are hard at work and struggling with fever and fever should pay attention to the fact that they need such pure, natural and simple pleasures in order to maintain and enjoy life. The source of these rich pleasures is to make close and emotional contact with nature. Anyone can enjoy nature by looking at stars, flowers, trees and animals, but the depth of this pleasure is greater in a botanist or biologist. Regarding the relationship between short-term goals and stress, Hans Selie says that in explaining the general response to stress, it was shown that everything we do and everything that happens to us, and finally these three stages of adaptation energy in the body are limited and should be Consume it with calculated savings. This is the biological basis of human need to express themselves and achieve their goals. These three basic stages are surprise (warning reaction), mastery (resistance stage), fatigue, and gradually moving to the stage of calm and repeating the same stages or reaching the final stage, which is death. Man was created to go through these stages. Therefore, it is necessary for him to prepare himself to go through them, and he does not miss any of these stages, to use each stage and enjoy it to the fullest, and at the same time to save his energy as much as possible.

2- Long-term goals

Long-term goals are set for future satisfaction. They do not currently have much impact on our well-being, health and comfort, but on the contrary, in most cases, they are in conflict with them. Sally says that every person, whether he believes in the existence of a creator for this universe or not, understands that his goals must go beyond the moments and to achieve it. Give up some momentary goals as well. To achieve long-term goals, we must work and learn how to choose between the paths that stand before us. But the main drawback is that the goals must be clarified precisely and we must build a way of life based on it so that we do not fall into the inevitable conflict between the present and the future. Long-term goals are essentially social, so striving for the future is an effort to create an atmosphere of happiness. These goals can put us on the path to an active, meaningful, happy, and long life, and keep us away from the unnecessary effects and harms of stress caused by militancy, deprivation, and insecurity. Seliyeh goes on to say that some people find these future goals in the accumulation of wealth and power, and some in religion and philosophy. A group also despairs of the future and wanders and wonders, spend their time from day to day and use methods such as wandering, constant travel, overwork or resorting to alcohol to divert their attention from the future. Keep away. A number of people also dedicate themselves to others and justify their future based on love, kindness and goodness. From what has been said about the relationship between long-term goals, Selie concludes that a clear and realistic pattern of adjustment and behavior that does not fit the personality structure results in mental illness, deprivation, feelings of insecurity and aimlessness, and migraine headaches. Stomach and intestinal ulcers, heart attacks, vascular disorders, high blood pressure, suicide or just a sad and bitter life.

3- The ultimate goal

Seliyeh believes that the ultimate goal of human beings is to flourish as much as possible. Based on the construction of his existence, this is the destination that should be the basis of all his activities. If a person strives to achieve his absolute existence and creation or to be in harmony with nature and society, it is necessary to strike a balance between his short-term and long-term goals. It means creating a kind of balance between planting and reaping in a way that his existence allows. The goal, of course, is not to avoid stress altogether. This is neither possible nor desirable. Because stress is a part of life and a natural product of our existence and environment, we have no reason to eliminate stress, but in order for a human being to be able to reach the level of his existential value to flourish and realize it, it is necessary to first know the desired level of stress. And then use the stored energy for compatibility in a desirable and beneficial way. Of course, to the extent that it corresponds to the physical and mental capacity of the person.

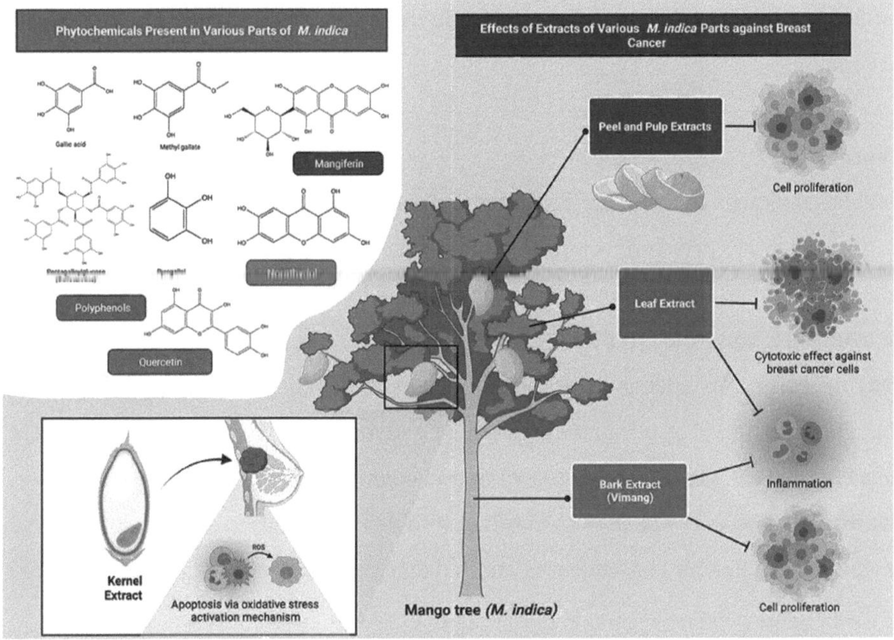

Figure 33. Mangifera indica: hopeful medicinal plant for breast cancer

The relationship between stress and illness

Everyone is attacked from time to time by cancer cells, which often destroy the immune system. But in conditions of severe anxiety, the peripheral part of the brain activates the hypothalamus, the body's thermostat. The hypothalamus paralyzes the immune system by triggering a war or flight response, increasing the chances of cancer cells multiplying. Doctors know for documented reasons that suppressed immune systems allow cancer cells to grow. In one particular case, doctors replaced a defective kidney with a healthy one. Depending on the operating conditions, the patient was injected with drugs that disrupted his immune system. A few days later, a tumor grew on the patient's chest. Further examination revealed that the patient's new kidney had malignant precellular cells. Cancer cells had spread from the kidneys to the lungs. The doctor immediately stopped taking drugs that neutralized the immune system, and within a few days there was no sign of cancer in the patient. Doctors explained that the new kidney may have cancer cells in it, and that the body stopped taking anti-inflammatory drugs. The new kidney was destroyed. But cancer cells were no longer external.

Worry

Feeling anxious occurs while confronting an imaginary or real threatening factor, during which the person develops tragic imaginary plays and stories in his mind and imagines the consequences in his mind and tries to do so mentally. From confrontation or avoidance, solve the problem.

On the child: An attempt to solve a problem in which a sequence of disturbing thoughts is triggered by a frightening stimulus and mental activity is pursued to prevent an adverse event. He considers anxiety to be a cognitive mechanism of avoidance.

Matthews: Unsuccessful attempt to solve a problem that leads to a continuous mental review of threatening consequences and in some cases creates mental scenarios and actively hinders the successful solution of the problem.

The difference between anxiety and anxiety: Anxiety is a major symptom in most areas of mental pathology, especially anxiety disorders such as generalized anxiety disorder, unconsciousness and practical obsession. Matthews sees anxiety as the result of anxiety, and when the problem is considered uncontrollable, he calls it the anxiety-anxiety spiral. Morris and Libert consider anxiety to be multidimensional and point to its emotional (physiological) and cognitive (anxiety) aspects. Sarason divides cognition in anxious people into areas of concern and inappropriate thinking. Burkok refers to trait anxiety as the time spent worrying, and considers anxiety to be the main construct of trait anxiety. But Brintz and Graham believe in the independence of anxiety from worry, and the main characteristic of worry is the focus on the problem.

The difference between fear and anxiety: Fear is an unpleasant feeling that occurs in response to a real danger. But worry is a frightening thought in the absence of real danger.

The difference between worry and obsessive thoughts: Worry has a more verbal theme than obsessive thoughts. Obsessive thoughts are more visual. Anxiety is rated as more real, less involuntary, and harder to get rid of, more distracting, and longer lasting.

The difference between worry and spontaneous thoughts: Spontaneous thoughts occur quickly, have a spontaneous aspect, and are expressed verbally or visually. The theme of thoughts is specific to each disorder. For example, in social fear, it is related to the fear of negative evaluation by others. Spontaneous thoughts are more reflective, but worry requires more attention. Anxiety occurs as a chain of thoughts that has an emotional theme. In fact, when anxiety occurs, one can think of it as a warning, a warning that forces us to look for unfinished problems in our lives by examining the events around us and our thoughts. So, it worries us to deal with the burden of unsuccessful and unresolved issues in our lives. Anxiety becomes traumatic when a person does not have sufficient skills to solve the problem and the problem of anxiety joins the group of chronic and unresolved problems in our lives. Contrary to popular belief that worry is a feeling, worrying is a kind of thinking, and for this reason, worrying may be a more telling alternative to worrying. It is worth noting that little independent research has been done in the psychological literature on anxiety. This lack of attention is due to the inappropriate definition of anxiety and the similarity of anxiety and worry.

The main feature of concern

A) Uncontrollability: The study showed that uncontrollability is the main feature of anxiety after onset. The hypothesis of uncontrollability has been confirmed by the population with concern. In the study by Berkowck et al., People who experienced higher levels of anxiety on a daily basis had great difficulty ignoring their anxieties and negative thoughts. But those who reported less anxiety believed that they were able to ignore or control unwanted thoughts in various ways.

B) Unwanted thoughts: Concerned people have significantly more disturbing and negative cognitive activities as well as more daily routine and less ability to control attention compared to non-concerned or normal people, an important factor that distinguishes the concerned group from normal groups. Unwanted thoughts are negative. What matters in a set of unwanted thoughts is not whether the thoughts are positive or negative, but how the person responds or copes with the onslaught of these thoughts in the mind and how the person copes with it and, in their opinion, pays attention to a Thinking and engaging the mind or ignoring it may be far more important than the positive or negative characteristics of thought.

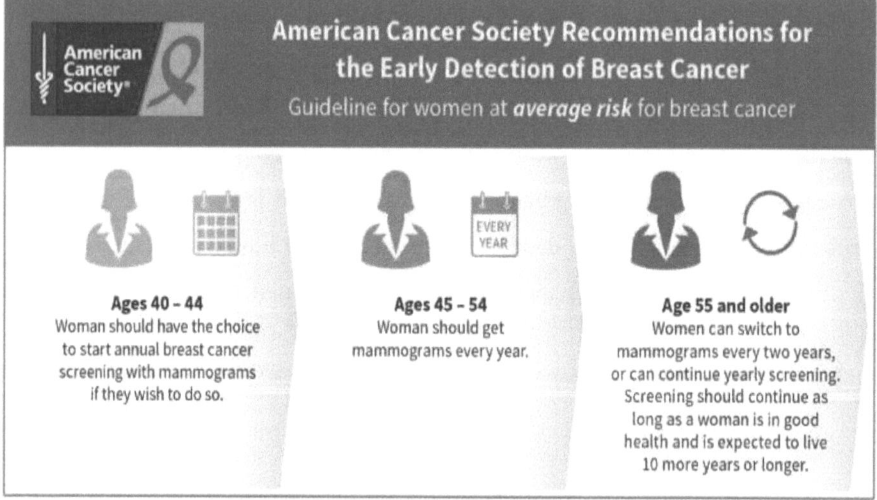

Figure 34. Emotional stress can cause Breast Cancer

Types of worries

1- Catastrophic worry: The main feature is the exaggerated definition and explanation of the problem and it occurs when a person's thoughts about a potential form are constantly superior, psychologists call this concern a "but" "if" method.

2- Hesitant and confused state of worry: It is characterized by obvious inability to make decisions and the result is a longer duration of worry. In another classification, anxiety is divided into two types, one and two.

- ✓ Type 1 Concern: Concern about an issue that is likely to occur to the individual.
- ✓ The second type of worry is worrying about worrying (I'm afraid this worry will drive me crazy).

Causes of concern

1- Personality: People who are banned and prevented in childhood are more prone to anxiety and GAD in adulthood. Personality traits such as emotional feelings and shyness make you more anxious.

2-Behavior/Learned: Our thinking habits are influenced by family and environmental factors. The tendency to visualize worry can train our minds to become accustomed to worry.

3- Family: Parents' role model can be effective in developing anxiety.

4- Brain biochemistry: Lack of chemicals in the brain is effective in causing anxiety and worry.

5- Social and cultural factors.

Personality traits of concerned people

1- Control center: People with high external control center have the highest vulnerability to fall into the abyss of the vicious cycle of "anxiety-worry".

2- Self-esteem and perfectionism: People with chronic anxiety have low self-esteem in solving problems and people with chronic anxiety usually have an avoidant and perfect personality.

3- Doubt and hesitation: People who are worried have an extreme need for evidence and reason to make a decision.

4- Concentration of mind and sleep: Worry is related to the frequency of annoying and negative thoughts. They have relatively higher levels of disturbed and scary sleep.

Areas of concern

- ✓ Anxious events often involve more failure than annoyance.
- ✓ Thinking about the future is often more frustrating than thinking about the past.
- ✓ Everyone's level of concern is commensurate with his experiences and his personality.

Transformation of anxiety in children

Fear of worries depends on the perception and understanding and anticipation of threats, all of which are related to cognitive abilities. This cognitive question seems to be acquired in children after the age of 7 (objective operation). Therefore, it can be argued that fear and anxiety are more prevalent among children with high levels of cognitive development. Wells' metacognitive model of the etiology of anxiety (positive and negative beliefs about anxiety) states that both positive and negative beliefs about anxiety are effective in the pathological development of anxiety. People who have positive beliefs about worrying, consider worrying as helping to solve a problem, increase motivation, etc. These beliefs help maintain and strengthen anxiety. Negative beliefs about anxiety exacerbate natural and pathological anxiety, which includes anxiety, anxiety, and GAD.

Morbid concern

1- Style: If this concern is directed at itself, it produces depression and severe physical illness such as cancer, and if it is directed at others, it produces aggression and aggression.

2- General: In a study on pathological and non-pathological concerns, these results have been reached. High pathological scores in clinical groups are associated with GAD, and high scores of pathological anxieties in non-clinical groups are associated with characteristic anxiety, increased self-awareness, low self-esteem, high depression, and so on.

3- Chelminsky: Pathological anxiety scores in GAD and obsessive-compulsive patients are higher than other anxiety disorders. Pathological anxiety scores are also significantly higher in GAD than in depression.

Physical effects of worry

Decreased resistance of the human body to infections, psychological stimuli stimulate the regulatory processes of the central nervous system. Cortisol secretion suppresses the immune system, and anxiety is directly related to physicality and insomnia.

The relationship between worry and compatibility

Anxiety is adaptive when it has the following three conditions:

- ✓ Warning to identify the threat.
- ✓ The direction of adaptive behavior and adaptation against threatening factors.
- ✓ Preparing the person to deal with threatening factors.

People who are concerned about finding successful solutions to weak problems are very strong at defining problems.

Types of processes to deal with the perception of threat

1- Information review: Search for more information about the threatening factor that leads to negative psychological and physical factors.

2- Ignorance method: It means trying to avoid information about the threatening factor of gender and concern. Women are seen as those who express greater ear, need more security, and lower power of representation. But men in the face of a similar situation perceive more anger and greater power of domination. In the case of women, the role of factors such as lower social status and inability to control things, as well as brain biochemistry (having low levels of the anxiety-controlling chemical) are mentioned.

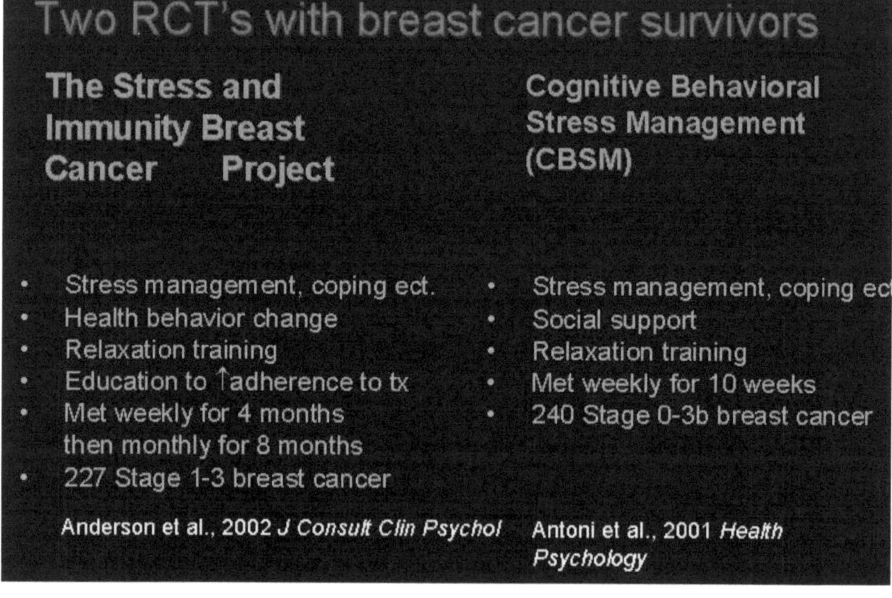

Figure 35. Healing the Mind Healing the Body Coping with

Concern models

Berkock Theory

1- Learning theory: Neutral stimulus due to association with fear stimulus based on the principle of association and classical conditioning alone causes the person to be afraid of these annoying conditioned stimuli and such reactions are strengthened by reducing the level of fear.

2- Cognitive processes: Berkuk worries are considered as an attempt to prevent and then avoid the occurrence of countless possible future consequences.

3- Self-esteem: self-assessment, which leads to the perception of the difference between self-idealism and the real self. This discrepancy is a cause for concern. The complexity, the lack of relevant empirical evidence, the incoherence of the elements of the theory, and the paradox that anxiety is associated with increased anxiety, but avoidant behavior is associated with decreased anxiety.

Talis and Isik theory

Talis and Isaac worked on the positive aspects of concern. The main functions of concern in their view are: alarm function, guidance function, preparedness function.

Determinants of threat value from the perspective of Talis and Isik

- ✓ The possibility of mentally occurring an annoying event.
- ✓ The imminence of the event mentally.
- ✓ Perception of the suffering of the event.
- ✓ Understanding strategies to overcome the event after the occurrence.

Dimensions that determine the intensity of the stress stimulus

- ✓ The importance of interests or goals whose development is likely to be stopped by an accident.
- ✓ Number of stopped goals.
- ✓ Severe deprivation.

Three stages of concern in the theory of Talis and Isik

- ✓ (Threat assessment) includes the damage to the person, the imminence of the threat, the probability of occurrence and estimating the efficiency of the person.
- ✓ (Stimulating and activating anxiety) The person responds to the components of the first stage.
- ✓ The person does not succeed by providing the correct response to the threat (by adopting incorrect problem-solving methods). As a result, the mentality of threat is reinforced and established, and a state of concern is created.

Model Barlow

Barlochenin argues that extreme anxiety is the result of several complex events:

1- Some situations with unexplained arousal led to the recall of anxiety statements stored in memory and create a negative emotional state.

2- Negative emotion shifts the attention from the external environment to the internal environment and causes it to focus on internal evaluation.

3- Attention and focus on self-evaluation leads to increased internal arousal.

4 - Increased activity and arousal of cognitive schema causes a state of all-round and excessive alertness, during which the person becomes extremely accurate to his own cognitive schema, and this state causes a hypothetical inability to predict and control events. The future as well as hypersensitivity and attention are limited. Limited attention is very important because it prevents attention from being drawn to irrelevant external events.

5- Activation of the schema creates hypersensitivity to fear.

6- Worry leads to inactivity, which increases the negative emotion, and as a result, these events occur in a new form.

Metacognitive model of concern

The metacognitive model of anxiety distinguishes between positive and negative beliefs about anxiety. Positive beliefs about anxiety lead to the use of anxiety as a coping strategy, while negative beliefs lead to a negative evaluation of anxiety (transcendence). Positive beliefs about anxiety are common and not necessarily harmful. However, the activity of metacognitive and related meta-negative beliefs is involved in the development of generalized anxiety disorder. While the existence of positive beliefs is not in itself problematic, using anxiety as a persistent coping strategy is problematic as it may interfere with other useful and adaptive self-regulatory processes. For example, stress following exposure to stress may interfere with the effectiveness of processing and controlling unwanted thoughts. Unwanted thoughts usually occur in the form of the question "what happens" and sometimes as negative images such as an image of being involved in an accident. The trigger activates positive metacognitive beliefs about worry as a means of counteracting the occurrence of an unintended thought event. Examples of positive beliefs are: "If I'm worried about all the possibilities, I can avoid failure," "Worrying about mistakes means I'm ready."

Type I anxiety is often a verbal process that involves a series of catastrophic and imaginative responses and is associated with emotional changes. The person becomes more anxious when the negative consequences are processed and experiences less anxiety when the goal of coping strategies is met. Type 1 anxiety usually persists until the person achieves the goal of anxiety. This is often pointed out by an emotion that indicates that the person is able to cope or an assessment that shows the most results and consequences are being considered. Concerns may also be replaced by situationally disturbed demands. Negative beliefs about anxiety become active during periods of anxiety in pathological anxiety states such as generalized anxiety disorder. These negative beliefs have two areas of content: uncontrollable and dangerous. A person with generalized anxiety disorder believes that anxiety is uncontrollable and potentially dangerous to physical, psychological, or social well-being. Examples of these beliefs are: "Worry is uncontrollable, I will lose my mind because of worry." A person who activates these beliefs leads to the development of negative interpretations of anxiety (transgression) and negative interpretations of emotional symptoms as a sign of loss of control or physical or psychological catastrophe, resulting in increased anxiety and feelings of threat. Thus, it becomes very difficult for the person to achieve an inner state that the person is coping (because the anxiety has not decreased) and thus it becomes more impossible to stop the symptoms of worry. There are two other mechanisms that lead to the activity and persistence of pathological anxiety.

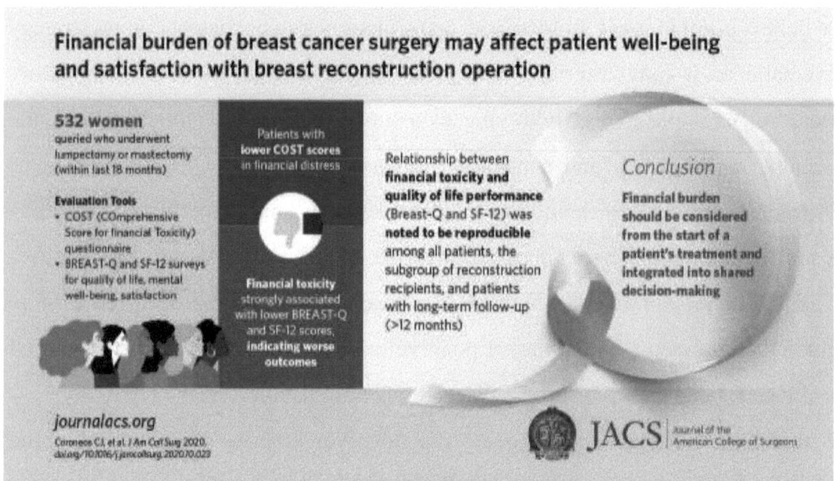

Figure 36. Financial distress associated with breast cancer surgery negatively impacts psychological

First, behaviors such as seeking reassurance and avoiding situations that trigger unwanted thoughts maintain negative beliefs about lack of control and risk. This is because one relies on external factors to control thoughts or avoids the size of the picture and the opportunities that show that worry is harmless.

Second, thought control strategies that seek to suppress thought that can trigger anxiety. This is anti-belief and leads to a greater awareness of the concept of concern, highlighting the need for concern and beliefs about their uncontrollability. In addition, the person does not interrupt the activated worry process. This is because it is inconsistent with beliefs about the need to worry and beliefs about uncontrollability.

Thus, an inconsistent thought control model is developed because its purpose is to try to remove the content of the thought from consciousness (for example, do not think about failure) until it decides not to engage in type I anxiety in response to unwanted thought. This model prevents the person from revealing that the worrying process is controllable, however, even if the anxiety is stopped, it protects the person from revealing that the worry is harmful.

Concern Avoidance Model

The model of anxiety avoidance and disseminated anxiety disorder is based on Moore's two-stage theory of fear and is also derived from the emotional processing of Foa and Kozak. According to the anxiety avoidance model, anxiety is based on verbal language intellectual activity that prevents clear mental imagery, physical participation, and emotional activation.

This prevents physical experience and emotional activation. This inhibition of physical and emotional experience prevents the emotional processing of fear, which is theoretically a barrier to suppression. In other words, increasing emotional and physical experience can lead to signs of effective emotional processing. The resulting suppression or silence may be exposed to a full range of fear symptoms, such as the stimulus itself, the response to stimuli in addition to the meaning behind the fear. Anxiety can therefore be seen as a fruitless cognitive effort to solve a problem and eliminate a perceived threat, while at the same time avoiding disgusting emotional and physical experiences that occur naturally during the fear-making process. he does. In addition, the experience of anxiety is negatively reinforced. According to the anxiety avoidance model, the catastrophic mental imagery created during the anxiety processing is replaced by less distressing thoughts and physically by the use of verbal verbal activity. Anxiety is thus negatively reinforced by the displacement of terrifying images. In addition, anxiety is reinforced by positive beliefs such as the belief that worry is useful and effective in problem solving, motivational performance, and avoiding negative consequences in the future. Positive beliefs are reinforced when negative events do not occur in the future or are effectively managed. So, they lead to more concern.

Dealing with worries

1. **Prescribing controlled anxiety:** Voluntarily paying for anxiety for a short period of time, this process is called work janissary or anxiety processing.

2. **Reducing the duration of worry by increasing the speed of thinking:** Since concerned people resist making quick decisions, so speeding up the decision-making process will be a constructive and useful action.

3. **Reducing anxiety and level of arousal:** The use of sedation methods in this field is recommended.

4. **Limiting the type of issues (mental preoccupations):** It means that we limit the concerned people to solvable issues. Because people who are worried cannot distinguish between previously solvable and unsolvable problems, so when people are presented with an unsolvable problem, instead of stopping their efforts, they continue to struggle mentally to find a solution.

5. **Positive mental activity:** Badley believes that worry requires the use of a working memory system. Therefore, engaging people in work that requires active and optimal use of memory is effective. As uninterrupted mental activity increases, the likelihood of disturbing and disturbing thoughts decreases. Strengthening the ability to solve mental-behavioral problems consists of 5 parts: orienting towards the problem, defining the problem, producing reasons, making decisions and applying solutions.

6. **Increased perceived self-efficacy:** Increased self-confidence, which increases the individual's ability to make decisions.

7. **Increasing a person's mental readiness:** If a person cannot control stressful stimuli, but if he can predict it, he will reduce the intensity of stress.

8. **Correcting people's moods:** Depressed and anxious moods increase anxiety. With regular exercise and fitness, the brain alters chemical levels such as serotonin, which improves mood.

Feeling lonely

Feeling lonely by many definitions is a distressing experience that leads to severe psychological and physical problems. Feelings of loneliness are associated with suicide, substance abuse, gloom and misery, and multiple physical illnesses. Statistics show that one in four people suffers from feelings of loneliness. Therefore, effective recognition and evaluation of loneliness is important. Research on loneliness over the past two decades reveals two major perspectives on loneliness. In the first view, the feeling of loneliness is considered as a single and integrated state that is caused by shortcomings in various relationships. That is, feeling lonely in different situations has a single cause, differing only in intensity. Previously valid tools for feeling lonely, such as the UCLA 20-item scale. Based on this approach, with a one-dimensional look, they measure the feeling of loneliness. In the second view, loneliness is a multidimensional phenomenon that varies in severity, causes and conditions. Although this view considers different types of feelings of loneliness to have a common core, it emphasizes that the consequences associated with defects in different relationships, such as feelings of loneliness in specific areas of communication, are qualitatively different. Proponents of this approach argue that this kind of conceptualization of loneliness reflects diverse and distinct experiences of loneliness.

For example, there are qualitative differences between the feeling of loneliness of a growing teenager and the transition to adulthood and the feeling of loneliness of an adult who has lost his wife. Critics of the one-dimensional approach to loneliness argue that general scales are unable to fully capture the multifactorial nature of loneliness. Following these criticisms, Weiss first distinguished social loneliness from emotional loneliness in 1973 in order to determine the nature of the dimensions of loneliness. Based on this distinction, the feeling of emotional loneliness means insufficient attachment to family, friends and close people, while the feeling of social loneliness comes from an insufficient number of friendships.

The feeling of loneliness is as old as human life, and sometimes it is even considered a natural aspect of human life and the result of his awareness of his exile in the world and his inevitable death, but it was not practically addressed until the early twentieth century. The first written article on this subject was written by Zilburg in 1938. This topic was the subject of mainly psychoanalytic research in the two decades of 1950-60 and was introduced as an independent entry in "Psychological Abstracts" from the mid-1970s and has been a field of research in social and clinical psychology ever since. In our Iranian culture, the issue of loneliness and its positive and negative consequences have been raised for a long time.

In Islamic culture of Iran, solitude, i'tikaaf and self-calculation have been emphasized. Although "Abraham Maslow" describes one of the hallmarks of self-fulfilling prophecies as the tendency to solitude and loneliness, what we mean here is loneliness, not loneliness in the full sense of the word, and loneliness other than loneliness. That is, although loneliness can be a desirable trait of self-fulfilling prophecies, the feeling of loneliness has many negative consequences. One of the necessities of our existence is the need to associate and associate with others. The source of this necessity is our social life. Some people who run away from socializing and spend most of their time alone may imagine a flaw in their thinking and existence that exacerbates the isolation. If solitude and isolation reduce the spiritual and intellectual powers, and if it is like imprisonment, forced and continuous, it is the most severe rewards and the most painful torments. Those who run away from the crowd do not dislike socializing, but fear the repetition of bitter experiences and past misfortunes.

For example, they cannot see that others are smarter and more worthy than them, or they cannot compete and fight with others in speech and action, or they have taken the method of isolation and loneliness at home from their parents and have become accustomed to it. Their consolation brings reasons for good isolation and expediency, and whether they like it or not, they convince themselves that the suffering of loneliness is less than the suffering of companionship. Feeling lonely is not the only product of modern urban life and the advancement of technology. From ancient times the attention has been paid to the human mind.

Although the feeling of loneliness has been considered by researchers as an experimental construct since the 1950s, its research began in the 1970s with the publication of Weiss's influential book, Feeling Lonely: The Experience of Emotional and Social Isolation. Loneliness is defined as a feeling of sadness and unhappiness combined with isolation: Loneliness is the feeling of being alone, cut off, or separated from others, accompanied by a feeling of not wanting to communicate, contact, or be close to others. Different theoretical perspectives have been put forward on the study of the formation and evolution of loneliness.

Some theoreticians, Sullivan and Balbi, have paid attention to the relationship between the child's parent and have considered the lack of proper communication with the child to be safe and satisfying as a factor in experiencing feelings of loneliness. The evolutionary perspective emphasizes that our ancestors at the beginning of history tried to live in groups and in relationships in order to protect themselves from environmental damage and in fact the feeling of loneliness it creates for them. Like a human baby who needs such connections to survive. As societies became more complex, communication itself became more important due to changing human needs. The human child with age needs to establish safe communication with other people, the background of which is formed in childhood.

Adolescence also creates its own sense of loneliness due to the special and unique features it brings. Adolescents can express their feelings, unlike children, who cannot talk about it with a proper understanding of loneliness. According to some experts, feeling lonely at this stage is normal. Adolescents at this stage, with their special cognitive characteristics such as hypothesis and self-centeredness, and with the thought that one day they will be separated from their parents, experience a kind of sadness that indicates their feeling of loneliness.

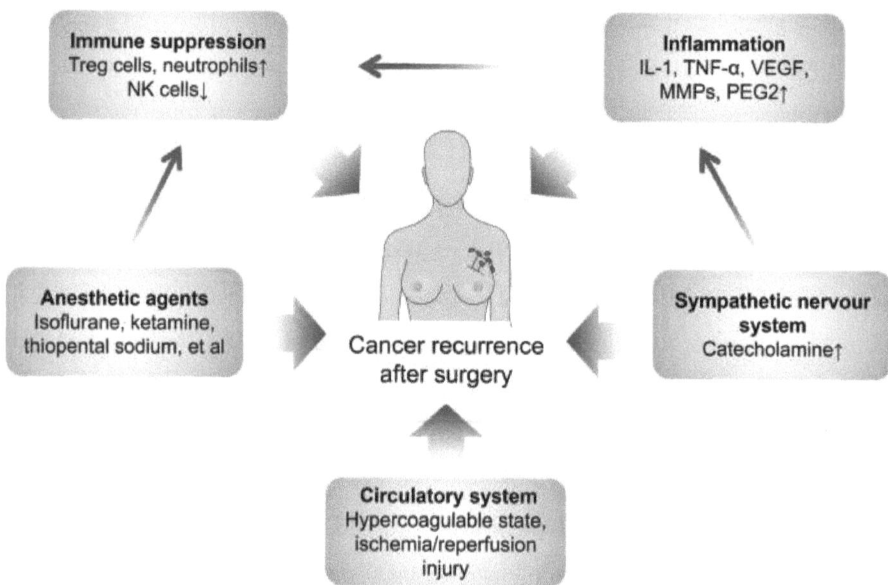

Figure 37. Surgical stress and cancer progression: the twisted tango

Types of loneliness

Alone can be divided into two categories with different sections of semiotics and therapeutic symptoms:

The first aspect of loneliness is the emotional isolation that results from the lack of important relationships in people's lives, such as death or divorce. The only way to cure loneliness. Finding important relationships with others in order to fill their vacancies. This loneliness is a memory of children's fears of leaving. This type of loneliness is often accompanied by pre-consciousness and anxiety that make people extremely sensitive to social cues, which can lead to misinterpretation or exaggeration of other people's tensions, both positive and negative. The second type of loneliness is called social isolation, which includes a lack of social network or lack of a place in the accepted society. In this type of loneliness, feelings about boredom, lack of focus, and feelings of being marginalized or rejected by peers are considered.

Theories of loneliness

Here is a brief overview of theories about loneliness:

1- Eric Fromm's theory

In the book Escape from Freedom, he writes: In the history of Western civilization, people have felt more lonely, meaningless and alienated by gaining more freedom. On the contrary, the less freedom people had, the greater their sense of belonging and security. Forum believes that people in the twentieth century have more freedom than in any other time, they feel more lonely, alienated and meaningless than the people of previous centuries.

2- Murray's artistic theory

According to Murray, the complex of simple isolation is experienced as the desire to be in small, warm, dark places that are safe and secluded. For example, a person may wish to stay under a blanket instead of getting out of bed in the morning. Murray refers to individuals as a complex of simple isolation and believes that individuals with this complex tend to be dependent on others, passive, and prone to safe behaviors.

3- Karen Horne

Horne refers to individuals only as "separate characters." Extremely strong characters tend to be relatively alone. They need to spend as much time alone as possible, and even sharing an experience like listening to music disturbs them.

4- Eric Erickson

The sixth stage of Ericsson's psychosocial stages is called intimacy versus isolation, which lasts from the end of adolescence until about age 35. During this time, we build close relationships with others and form a marital bond. People who are not able to have such intimacy in early adulthood feel isolated. They avoid social contact and reject others.

5- Abraham Maslow

Maslow considers the feeling of separation and solitude to be a feature of self-fulfilling prophecies, and believes that self-fulfilling prophecies can experience isolation without detrimental effects, and that they seem to need more alone than non-self-fulfilling prophecies.

Who are alone?

Men feel lonelier than women if they are not involved in a romantic relationship. Maybe because they have fewer options to satisfy their intimacy needs. Women feel lonelier in married life than their husbands, especially if they are not employed. Have recently moved or have young children, conditions that limit their access to the wider social network. If loneliness persists, it is associated with a variety of self-defeating attitudes and behaviors. Although some people are very lonely, most young people sometimes find themselves alone when trying to satisfy their unsatisfied desires for a relationship. As long as loneliness is not exhausting, it can encourage young people to find ways to enjoy loneliness and take this opportunity to deepen their self-awareness.

Treatment alone

Not surprisingly, group therapy has a great impact on treatment alone. Providing engagement with others reduces the degree of "marginalization." In addition, mutual help within the group reassures the individual and allows him to take the first steps to solve his problem. At the same time, he realizes that he is not alone. They also measure their progress by evaluating each other, and unlike emotional disorders, clients can report their progress positively.

Cancer and psychological factors

The causes of diseases are very numerous and complex. In addition, the relationships between these factors also play an important role in causing these diseases. In general, from the seventeenth century onwards, which is the period of scientific progress, especially in the field of medical science, there are three categories of recognizable factors in the description of diseases:

- ✓ Medical and biological factors, such as biochemical changes and cellular abnormalities.
- ✓ Social factors, such as life events.
- ✓ Psychological factors such as personality traits.

Based on these factors, a bio-social-psychological model is presented that emphasizes the interaction of biological, social and psychological factors in the development of diseases. In this approach, psychological and physiological factors are known as the cause of diseases and the social environment plays an important role in the occurrence of diseases by influencing psychological and physiological factors. Extensive research has been done on cancer and its psychosocial factors, the second leading cause of death in the United States since the mid-20th century.

In general, the relationship between cancer and psychological factors based on research conducted so far can be discussed in two areas. Factors that predispose to cancer and factors that affect the course of the disease. Although cancer is a psychosomatic disease, there is no evidence that psychological factors such as pain, failure, failure, depression, guilt, or any type of stress can cause any type of cancer.

Until now, there is no single and generally accepted cause for malignant tumors, no one is completely sure of the causes of cancer. Response to stressful events is affected by various factors. Among these factors are cognitive assessment, sense of control and social support. According to Lazarus, the factors that cause a stressful event to have a profound effect on one person while having little effect on the other are cognitive assessment factors. In his opinion, this evaluation is done in two primary and secondary stages. In a person's initial assessment of whether a particular situation is stressful?

Judges and in the secondary assessment the person assess his / her ability to deal with the stressful stimulus.

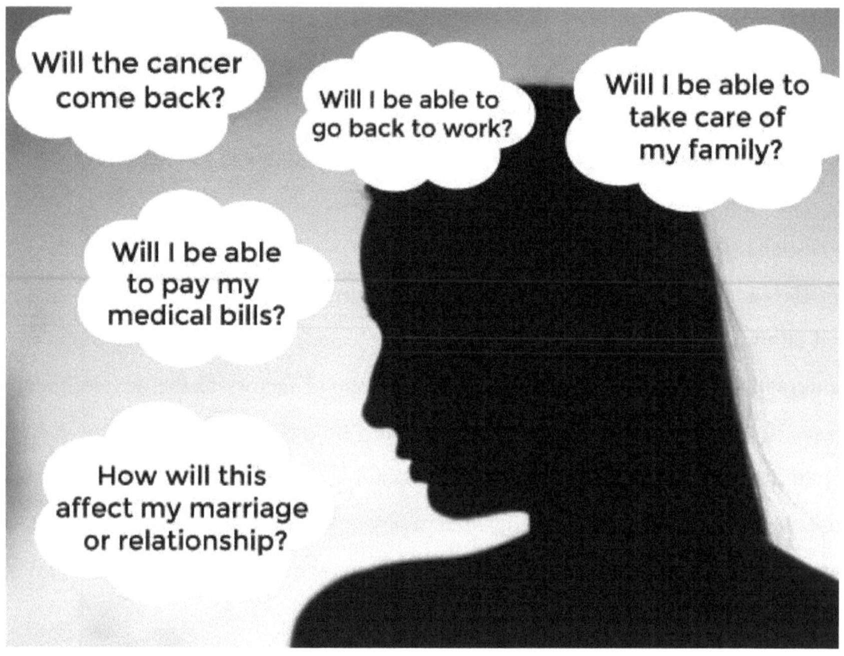

Figure 38. Managing Anxiety and Distress in Cancer Survivors

Feelings of control over the duration of a stressful event. Feeling in control over the course of a stressful event also reduces stress intensity, making emotional and social support more stressful. Research shows that people with broader social connections are less likely to develop malignant neoplasms than those without such connections. Researchers believe that the experience of stressful events significantly increases the consumption of substances such as tobacco and alcohol, the high consumption of which can be carcinogenic.

Cigarettes and diet have been identified as risk factors for cancer and the ways to exert such an effect are different. Cigarettes can be effective in the long-term target system of the immune system, reducing immune monitoring and possibly increasing the chances of tumor growth. Other functions of the immune system are also affected by smoking, and direct damage to the body system is possible. Dietary factors are also associated with cancer. The combination of alcohol and smoking has been shown to increase the risk of several types of cancer. Recent studies have also shown an association between alcohol consumption and cancer. Because psychosis and cancer have a complex relationship, according to research, there is no direct relationship between psychological factors and cancer progression.

In some cancers, the cancer cells have endocrine characteristics and may cause major depression in the patient by secreting steroids. For example, lung or pancreatic cancers. Also, difficult treatments and pain caused by the progression of the disease affect the psychological state of patients. It is a fact that people react differently to dangerous diseases such as cancer.

Research background on perceived stress and breast cancer

Qara Zibaei et al. In 2012 in a study entitled the effectiveness of semantic therapy on perceived stress and life expectancy in patients showed that semantic therapy method had a significant effect on reducing perceived stress and increasing life expectancy in patients and reduced perceptual stress. And increased life expectancy in patients.

Haddad et al. In 2010 in an article entitled "Study of the relationship between breast cancer incidence with stressful events and personality traits of individuals" that this study aims to investigate the relationship between breast cancer and personality and life stress as a beginning Has been performed in the incidence of this cancer. This is a descriptive cross-sectional study in which 155 female patients aged 20-70 years, referred to Haft Tir Hospital and Tehran Cancer Institute during 7 months in 2006 were studied. The level of education of the subjects was at least fifth elementary and in two groups of women with breast cancer, 85 people and 70 non-infected women were placed. Data collection was performed using two questionnaires of stressful life events of Pickle and Cloninger personality questionnaire. Both groups were evaluated in terms of personality traits and life stresses. Data were analyzed using descriptive statistics, Mann-Whitney and t-tests in SPSS 17 software.

Finally, we understand that there is a relationship between life events, high-risk life events and the severity of each of them with the incidence of breast cancer. There is also a link between the two personality traits of perseverance and more self-aggrandizement, which to some extent indicate the obsessive traits and, of course, spiritualism of individuals, with the incidence of breast cancer. It has been suggested that more extensive studies in this area are recommended.

Ebrahimi et al. In 2009 in examining the relationship between adverse events and the incidence of breast cancer in patients referred to the Breast Diseases Center showed that there was a relationship between the history of physical or mental illness of the spouse, the number of adverse events (stressful and worrying events) and child unemployment with breast cancer There is significance. However, there is no significant relationship between the cumulative effect of adverse events and their severity and also after multivariate analysis between their number and this disease.

Yavar et al. In 2006 in an article examined the risk factors related to breast cancer in women referred to Shohada Tajrish Hospital in Tehran and in the results of their research reported that the variables of marital status (singleness), family history, radiographic history from the chest before the age of 30, the low number of live births, the high age of the mother in the first live birth, menopause and the use of birth control pills were identified as important risk factors for breast cancer.

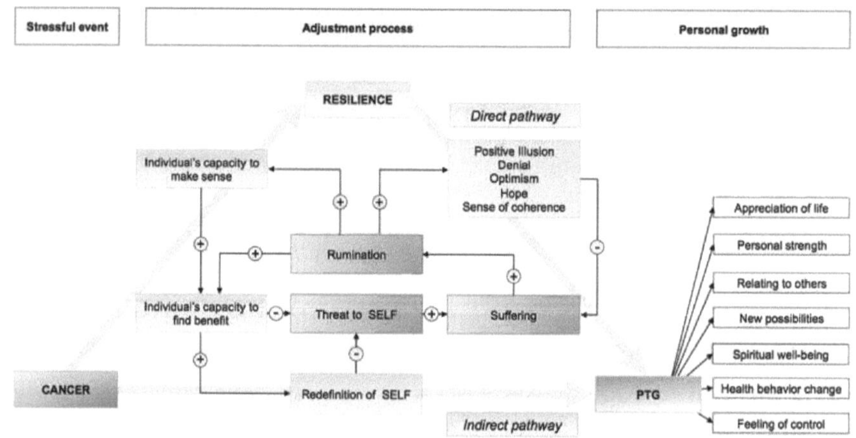

Figure 39. Resilience in Cancer Patients

Taleghani in 2005 in a study entitled How to adapt to the disease in 20 patients with breast cancer, found that adaptation to breast cancer in women has a positive evolutionary trend and is more in line with the disease. The strategies that these women used to adapt to their illness included religious strategy, thinking about the illness, accepting the truth of the illness and social and cultural factors, and finally social support. Most of the applied strategies by Iranian women were positive. Religious belief played an important role in these women.

Bakhtiari et al. In 2003 in an article entitled Study of the relationship between demographic, social characteristics and lifestyle with breast cancer in women showed that breast cancer is one of the most common cancers in women. Identifying risk factors for this cancer through preventive strategies reduces the risk of developing this disease. The aim of this study was to determine the relationship between some demographic, social and lifestyle characteristics with breast cancer. The method of study was that in this case-control study was performed in Shahid Rajaei Chemotherapy-Radiotherapy Center in Babolsar. 72 patients with breast cancer and 85 healthy women who were identical in age and place of residence (as a control group) were included in the study by convenience sampling method. Chi-square and t-test were used for statistical analysis. The results of this study showed that there is a significant relationship between breast cancer and economic, social, menarche age, family history of breast cancer and other cancers in 1st and 2nd degree relatives, history of breast trauma, smoking or passive contact with cigarettes, diseases Chronic internal use, low physical activity, stressful life and high body mass index, but there is a significant relationship between breast cancer and pregnancy variables, age of first pregnancy, number of abortions, lactation, OCP use, history of benign breast diseases, biopsy There were no breasts or menopausal age. Therefore, the final conclusion is that this study supports the fact that the family history of breast cancer, stressful life, the presence of chronic internal diseases, obesity, economic status, low social status are important factors in breast cancer. Therefore, this study suggests that lifestyle modifications such as smoking cessation, regular exercise and screening tests can reduce the risk of breast cancer.

In a 2008 review, Rinat, Libert, and John concluded that external factors such as stress, long-term anxiety, and social support have a significant effect on the components of the immune system that influence the onset or course of cancer. They also stated that the relationship between psychological factors and cancer is very complex and includes several biological, psychological and social systems.

In a 2002 study entitled The Relationship between Stressful Events in Breast Cancer Patients, Mansell et al. Showed that there was a significant difference between stressors and breast cancer patients in both normal and normal groups. So that the amount of perceived stress by patients was 2.7 times higher than normal people. Patients also considered many events that were not worrying and stressful for ordinary people as stressful events.

Wisplar, Reinart Wilbert In 2001, a study of 51 women with malignant breast cancer, 71 women with benign breast glands and 30 women in the control group using the Center for Control and Intimate Relationships questionnaire (married couple) found that women with cancer Breasts have less internal control than others and their health depends on luck. They also want less intimacy and closeness and there is a big distance between them, their couple and their family. Rinat, Libert, and John Derwy concluded in studies that external factors such as stress, depression, or social support have a significant effect on the components of the immune system that influence the onset or course of cancer. In their view, the relationship between psychological factors and cancer is very complex and includes the interaction of several biological, psychological and even social systems with each other.

In a 1999 prospective study, Hagen List listed women who referred to an outpatient clinic for breast cancer screening. The results showed that women with interpersonal problems, despite the obvious impact of the problem on their lives, deny it and are at high risk for breast cancer. The ability to express anger as a mechanism for managing and controlling stressful events plays a role in reducing the risk of cancer, and the coping mechanism of denial increases the likelihood of being diagnosed with breast cancer in women. The findings also suggest Eisenhower's vaccination theory in 1983, which emphasizes the inhibitory effects of chronic stress on cancer cell formation and its adaptation to the effects of chronic stress in repetitive encounters. Eisenhower claims that adapting to chronic pressures has an immunizing effect on the body. Oscar and Anisman believe that acute stress leads to a decrease in catecholamines and an increase in ACTH, which leads to the synthesis and secretion of more hormones, thereby inhibiting and weakening the immune system. In chronic stress adaptation to biological mechanisms has been observed. In contrast, women who have experienced a loss (an acute stressors) and are greatly affected by it are classified as having a higher risk.

Hagen List in 1999 and Grosart-Matisk in Yugoslavia tested the subject in a psychosocial interview in 1985. Ten years later, in a study of their mortality rates, they found that those who died of cancer had high scores on the rationality / anti-emotional scale of the interview. Another cause of cancer-related mortality was long-term (rooted) frustration.

Grossart-Matissek, Eisenhower, and others conducted a prospective study by measuring depression, frustration, irritability, anger, rationality / anti-emotion, and the need for a personal relationship. They successfully and correctly predicted 71% of cancer cases and 63% of cancer deaths from preliminary data. Based on the information obtained from this study, Grossart-Mathisk, Eisenhower, and Veter introduced four personality types based on the type of stress response:

- ✓ Susceptible to cancer.
- ✓ Susceptible to cardiovascular disease.
- ✓ Two-sided (prone to mental disorders).
- ✓ Independent (healthy).

Matissek and Eisenhower later added two more brigades in 1990:

- ✓ Rational / anti-emotional tendencies (prone to depression).
- ✓ Anti-social tendencies (prone to crime and addiction).

In this division, type 1 (cancer-prone type) people are cooperative, very patient, calm, harmonious, daring, kind, have defensive and emotion-suppressing behavior, are not able to tolerate interpersonal stress, and in these situations feel helpless, they become frustrated and eventually depressed.

Bermund, Cowen, and Banson found in 1986 that women with breast cancer denied, internalized, and retaliated their emotions, especially anger, and believed in social norms for the control group. It is also very important for them to look good.

Forsen wrote in 1990 that women who experienced a severe absence six years before the tumor was diagnosed were 14 times more likely to develop breast cancer.

In a 1989 study of the specific characteristics of women with breast cancer, Todarloo et al. Found that cancer patients may have something in common with people with psychosomatic injuries. That is, limited imagery and daydreaming and difficulty in verbalizing emotions. Studies show that in women, waiting for acceptance indicates a poor or bad prognosis, and in men, frustration/ helplessness causes a recurrence.

In a study using path analysis, Eisenhower and others found that about half of the variance in cancer was due to personality / stress factors.

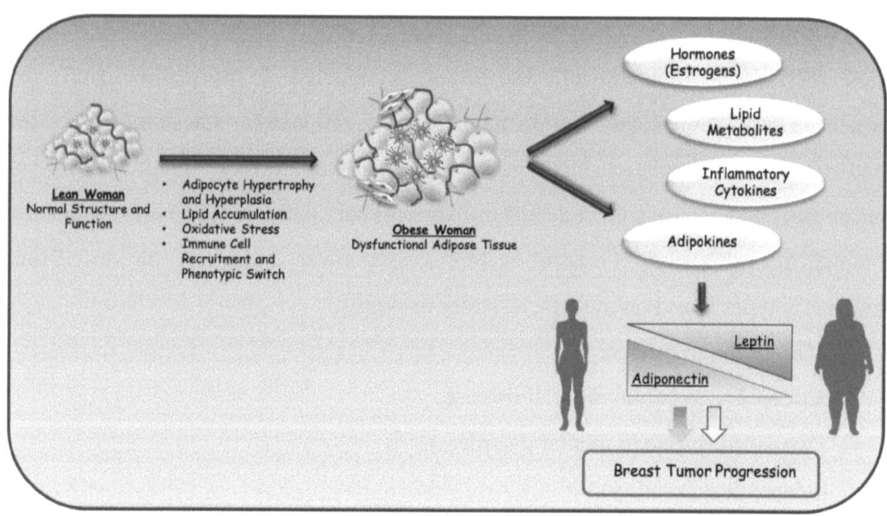

Figure 40. Obesity, Leptin and Breast Cancer: Epidemiological Evidence

Eisenhower Studies on educational and therapeutic interventions in cancer patients also show that these programs can increase the optimism of cancer patients and reduce feelings of hopelessness. In addition, an increase in the number of killer cells in the immune system of these people has been reported. Research also shows that people who are in the final stages of illness and who have been trained in the independence program have survived longer than those who have not.

Worry

Research similar to the present research is rare inside and outside the country. However, it goes back to cases of relatively similar research. Mohammadifard in 2012 in a study entitled Depression, anxiety and loneliness in patients with cancer, MS and its comparison with normal people, showed that both groups of patients have high rates of depression, anxiety and loneliness compared to Ordinary people had. They also showed that patients with MS had a greater sense of loneliness compared to cancer patients, but there was no significant difference in the variables of depression and anxiety. He also concluded that MS patients felt lonelier because they were mostly young (adolescents).

Bijari et al. In the study of the effectiveness of group therapy based on the hope therapy approach on increasing life expectancy in women with breast cancer. The title of the second goal is considered by quasi-experimental method (unequal control group design) and purposeful or available sampling and using Schneider hope and Beck depression tests. It is acknowledged that group therapy based on hope therapy approach Compared to the control group, it significantly increased life expectancy and decreased anxiety and depression in women.

However, in the study of Aladdin et al. Entitled The study of the effectiveness of group hope therapy on hope and mental health, one of the subscales of their study was the relationship between hope therapy and anxiety and insomnia and change in physical symptoms, a significant relationship between the two among 30 No subjects who were randomly assigned to the experimental and control groups were observed.

Bijari in her research showed that women with breast cancer are characterized by characteristics such as denial and suppression of emotions, especially anger, high surrender, non-expression, defensiveness and anti-irritability. This trait eventually leads to feelings of hopelessness and depression. Also, women with breast cancer are significantly more likely to use emotion-coping, avoidance, self-control, and avoidance coping techniques. The results of her research showed that hope therapy increases life expectancy in women with breast cancer and reduces depression in them.

Malekian et al. Concluded from their research that depression and anxiety are relatively high in cancer patients and affect performance, quality of life, length of hospital stay and even the outcome of cancer patients.

Abbas Portath studied the effect of mental imagery on the anxiety of female breast cancer patients at Imam Khomeini Hospital in Tehran. He found that this technique greatly reduces anxiety and stress.

A study found that leukemia patients use both emotion-based and problem-oriented coping. Anxiety has a negative and significant correlation with seeking social support and tendency to focus on emotion, but this relationship was significant with acceptance, submission and inhibition of positive emotion expression.

In the study of Ahmadi et al., The aim was to evaluate the physical, mental, psychological and social dimensions of quality of life during breast cancer undergoing chemotherapy. The results showed that improving the quality of life in women with breast cancer not only improves their survival, but also increases the quality of life and greater cohesion of the family structure.

Sobhanifard in a study entitled the effect of supportive psychotherapy in reducing mental disorder in women with breast cancer. The results of this study showed that the patients in the control group had more severe and profound symptoms compared to the experimental group.

In a study, Potagas et al. Examined the effect of anxiety and stressful life events on the recurrence rate of physical illness in Athens. The results of their study showed that high levels of anxiety were associated with the number and severity of reported stressful events.

A 2004 study by Hernandez-Reef et al. Found that message therapy immediately reduced depressed mood, anxiety, and anger in women with breast cancer. The longer-lasting effect of message therapy was to reduce the hostility of dopamine and serotonin and the immune system.

In a 2000 study by Foucault, Coca-Cola, Okmura, and Nakanishi, researchers looked at the effect of intervention methods on coping skills, stress management health education, and emotional-psychological support on cancer patients.

In this study, patients with the following conditions from a cancer treatment center in eastern Japan participated in the study. The method of their selection was based on a questionnaire and their mental status was assessed through the Anxiety Scale in the hospital. Considering the criteria for admission, 50 out of 151 eligible women participated in this study and were divided into two groups of intervention and control. The intervention groups consisted of 10-6 people under 90 minutes of training each week for 6 weeks. People were taught mental and planned visualization. Patients were asked to apply these skills according to the guidelines given in their daily lives and not to stop them during and after treatment. Psychological assessments of participating women were performed once at the beginning of the intervention and once in the sixth week and then in the sixth month of the intervention by the criteria for assessing stress and mental disorders. The results showed that the intervention group after the treatment, had a lower score for measuring anxiety and worry and a higher score in terms of psychological and emotional stability than the control group based on the study scale. The researchers concluded that despite the fact that six months had elapsed since the end of the treatment interventions, this place still had a reduction in the symptoms of psychological stress in patients during subsequent follow-ups. Therefore, they found such interventions easy, cost-effective and effective in treating mental and emotional disorders caused by breast cancer.

Bhutto et al. (2000) showed that suppression of cancer risk predictors was younger in women.

In their 1999 study of the quality of life of American women with breast cancer, Nortos et al. In Michigan found no significant association between demographic variables and disease such as age, education, marital status, and income quality of life.

Pump Anthony, Weisser, and Garson (1996) found in a study that social and psychological interventions enhance the coping skills of women with cancer and improve their emotional disturbances.

Loneliness

There has not been much direct and specific research on social loneliness and isolation, but there have been studies on some issues that are indirectly related to this issue, some of which are examined in this section.

Alizadeh Aghdam in 2012 in her article entitled "Study of the future hope among students and the factors affecting it using 24 six-item items, found the future hope of young people as moderate and that the effective variables are respectively, they were social cohesion, religiosity, cultural capital and social trust, these variables explained a total of 29% of the variance of the dependent variable.

 Kalantari et al. In 2012 in their research studied the social alienation of urban residents of Givi, one of the age groups was 33-20 years. The mean score of social alienation in the statistical sample was equal to 44.9 and in the mean and the relationship between age and social alienation was not significant. This means that young people also suffer from a significant amount of social alienation.

Soroush in 2012 in his research entitled "Individual and social responsibility, otherness and social trust: a study of adolescents in Shiraz" with a study of 291 adolescents aged 19-15 in Shiraz concluded that the level of responsibility as well as the level of social trust of adolescents in It was moderate, but their level of demand and other levels of trust in other groups was below average and low.

A 2013 study by Rotenberg et al found that loneliness was associated with many psychological characteristics of patients, such as low self-esteem, external evidence of success, embarrassment, shame, introversion, aggression, depression, stress, and anxiety.

The research findings of Margaret et al. Indicate that high levels of pessimism, introversion, loneliness and isolation, excessive expectation from others, and lack of responsibility for the emotional states of physically incurable patients are considered.

Deer in 2009 Some research has shown that girls feel lonelier than boys. Research shows that people who have persistent problems establishing and maintaining relationships with others and have difficulty satisfying their belonging needs have difficulty growing emotionally and socially, leading to psychological disturbances such as loneliness and depression. Therefore, recognizing and evaluating the characteristics of feeling lonely can be effective in helping mental health.

Bartrop et al. Studied 33 widowed couples and their control group and found that specific immune system indices were ten times weaker in the bereaved group. Subsequent studies have confirmed this finding.

Greer, Morris, Patin Gill, growing evidence suggests that frustration can play an important role in cancer vulnerability. Fifty-one women were admitted to the Rochester Clinic in New York for examination as soon as they arrived. Each of these women had previously identified suspicious cells in their cervix that they could definitively diagnose as cancer. The researchers found that 18 of the 51 women had experienced significant damage in the past six months, which they reacted to with feelings of hopelessness and loneliness. The rest of the women had not experienced such a life event. Eleven of the 18 disappointed people were diagnosed with cancer. Out of thirty-three, only eight had cancer. The difference between the two groups was statistically significant. Likewise, lack of meaning in life, job instability, and lack of plans for the future better predict who gets lung cancer than the amount of smoking. In contrast, breast cancer patients who responded with a fighting spirit instead of being patiently accepted had a better chance of surviving the disease five years later.

Barterp, Lockhart, Lazarus, Kiloway, and Penny are all examples of how depression, helplessness, hopelessness, loneliness, and stressful life events are related to changes in a person's immunity. Twenty-six spouses whose pair had died were followed up for six weeks after the death of their spouse. The bereaved group showed lower than normal T cell proliferation against antigens.

Irwin, Daniels, Bloom, Smith-Woniz In another study, it was found that natural killer cell activity was lower in women who had recently experienced major life events such as the death of their husband. The more depressed the woman, the weaker the NK and T cell function.

Carolyn Biddle-Thomas, a psychologist, found a statistical correlation between psychological factors and the health record of 1337 medical students who graduated between 1948 and 1964. She concluded that one of the most important prognostic factors in this group. Cancer, mental illness and suicide, lack of closeness and intimacy with parents and their negative perception of their family, and Leonard Seim in 1978 in a study conducted confirmed the importance of "social support" in physical and mental health. He found that mortality was two to three times higher among those who did not have close contact with others than among those with many associates. Research on animals also shows that even among them, social communication is of particular importance.

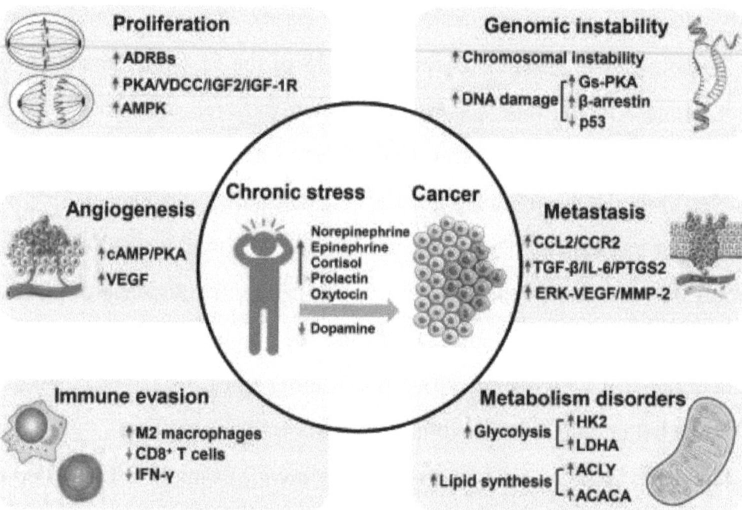

Figure 41. Cancer and stress: NextGen strategies

In one of these studies, which was performed on monkeys, it was observed that if a monkey was placed alone in front of a snake, it would be more nervous and restless than when confronted with it in a group of monkeys. Mice injected with cancer cells and isolated were dying much faster than mice that had social life.

A study of prisoners of war in Vietnam shows that communication between prisoners, even with visual cues and visual coders, has been a vital factor in their survival. Laboratory studies with animals have shown that by giving a specific system to stressful stimuli, their risks can be reduced. Some researchers exposed a group of monkeys to loud and annoying noises, but allowed another group to break the sound by pulling a chain. While both groups heard the same amount of sound, the blood in the group that was able to pull the chains contained less stress hormones. In this regard, mastering the situation had caused this noticeable difference. This is also true of humans and has been studied.

In a study of factory workers, Robert Karasik found that people who had little control over their jobs (such as workers who just closed the bottle or pressed a button to get a product out of the car) were more likely to do so. They suffer from heart disease rather than people who are independent in the quality, quantity and speed of their work. Workers such as telecommuters, restaurant workers, cashiers, and those who have the least ability to make independent decisions despite their high responsibilities are much more vulnerable to disease. He says the death toll in this group is about the percentage of deaths caused by excessive smoking or high blood cholesterol.

One of the biggest requirements for cancer research is longitudinal studies that are done before the onset of cancer symptoms in people. Obviously, such studies are difficult to do, because no one can predict whether or not people will develop malignant cancer. An ideal study is a study in which a large representative sample of seemingly healthy individuals is evaluated, then to determine which of them has cancer and whether its occurrence can be pre-collected by psychological data Predict cancer diagnosis or not? Follow up. Evidence suggests that psychological factors in cancer are still experimental. In most existing research, methodological limitations make definitive conclusions risky. The control group is inadequate or inadequate in many studies. They are ambiguous in the definition of psychological factors. They use psychological tests and questionnaires that are not well accredited or depend on the reassignment of patients who have already had cancer. Modifications to the research method may help clarify a number of questions that address the relationship between psychological factors and cancer.

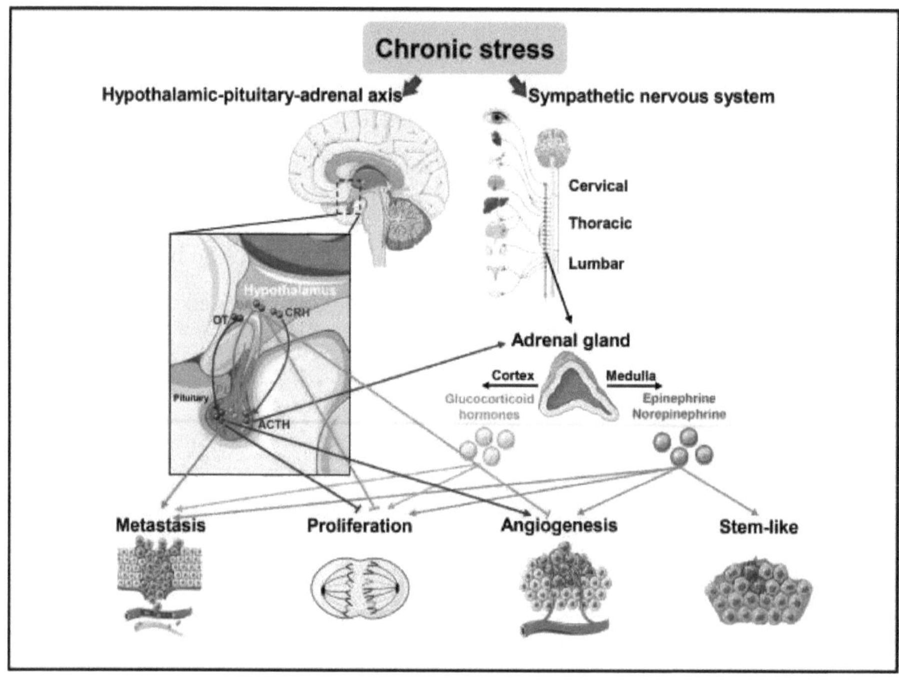

Figure 42. Cancer and stress: NextGen strategies

Reference

Aguilar-Ruiz JS, Riquelme JC, Toro M. Evolutionary Learning of Hierarchical Decision Rules, in IEEE Transactions on Systems 2003; 33(2): 324-34.

Andres C, Pena R, Sipper M. Designing Breast Cancer Diagnostic Systems via aHybrid Fuzzy-Genetic Methodology, IEEE International Fuzzy Systems Conference 1999; 1: 135-9.

Ashlaghi A, Pour Ebrahimi A, Ebrahimi M, Ahmad L. Using data mining techniques for prediction breast cancer recurrence, Iranian Journal of Breast Disease 2013; 5(4): 23-34.

Bewick M, Krause A. Her-2 Expression is a prognostic factor in patient with metastatic breast cancer treated with combination of High-dose cyclophosphamide, paclitaxel, Mitoxatrone and autologus Blood stem cell support. Bone Marrow transplantation 2001 Apr; 27(8): 847-53.

Bland KI, Verzerides MP, Copeland III EM. Breast In: Schwartz SI, Shires GT, Spencer FC, editors. Principles of surgery. 7 th ed. New York: McGraw Hill; 1999. P. 554-92.

Brodwicz I, Kandior O, Anti Her-2/Neu Antibody induces Apoptosis in Her-2/Neu overexpressing breast cancer cells independently from P53 status. British journal of cancer 2001 Nov; 85(11): 1764-70

Carr JA, Havstad S. The association of Her2 amplification with breast cancer recurrence. Archieves of surgery 2000 Des; 135(12): 1469- 74.

Cho HS, Mason K, Ramyor KK, Stanly AM, Gabell SB. Structure of the Extracellular region of Her-2 alone and in complex with herceptin Fab. Nature 2003 Feb 13; 421(6924): 756-60.

Colon E, Rayer JS, Gonzalez Keelan C, Climent peris C. Prevalence of steroied Receptor and Her-2/Neu in Breast biopsies of women living in puertorico. Puertorice health-sciences Journal 2002; 21(4): 299-303.

Daly JM, Bertagnolli M, Decosse JJ, Morton DM. Oncology in: Schwartz SI, Shires GT, Spencer FC, editors. Principles of surgery, 7th ed. New York: MC-Graw Hill; 1999. P. 308-9, 323.

Endo A, Shibata T, Tanaka H. Comparison of seven algorithms to predict breast cancer survival, Biomedical Soft Computing and Human Sciences 2008; 13(2): 6-11.

Fentiman IS. Fixed and modifiable risk factors for breast cancer. Int J Clin Prat 2001; 55(8): 527-30.

Ganji MF, Abadeh MS. Parallel Fuzzy Rule Learning Using an ACO-Based Algorithm for Medical Data Mining, IEEE Fifth. International conference on Bio InnspiredCompting: theories and Applications 2010; 573-81.

Gerber B, Krause A. Effectiveness of herceptin in patient with locally recurrence breast cancer after cardiac failure caused by sever cytotoxic pretreatment. Oncology 2001; 61(4): 271-4.

Herdy V. Education: a key factor in fighting breast cancer. New York: Inter press services 1998; 1.

Huge OF, Yamauch H. Circulating Her-2 extracellular domain as a prognostic factor with metastatic breast cancer. Clinical cancer research 2001 Sep; 7(9): 2605-7.

Iglehort JD, Kaelin CM. Breast. In: Tounsend courtney MJR, Beauchamp R.D, Mark Evers B. SABISTON text book of surgery. Philadelphia, pennesylvania: W.B. Saunders company; 2001. P. 568-90.

Iran Ministry of Health & Medical Education. Diseases management center, cancer office. Country report of cancer cases. Tehran: KelkZarrin Press 2004; 16. Sadeghnezhad F, NiknamiSh, Ghaffari M, Effect of health education methods on promoting breast self-examination (BSE), Journal of Birjand University of Medical Sciences 2009; 15(4): 38-48.

Iran Ministry of Health & Medical Education. Health deputy, Family Health office, adult health and women office. Primary report of breast cancer screening 1st ed. Tehran: Ministry of Health & Medical Education 2000; 18-36.

Jain R, Abraham A. A Comparative Study of Fuzzy Classification Methods on Breast Cancer Data, Australas Phys Eng Sci Med 2004; 27(4): 213-8.

Jain R, Mazumdar J. A Genetic Algorithm based Nearest Neighbor Classification to Breast Cancer Diagnosis, Australasian Physical & Engineering Sciences in Medicine 2003; 26(1):6-11.

Joen Sun H, Isola J, Lundin M, Salminen T, Holli K, Kataja V. Amplification of erb-b2 and erb-b2 expression are superior to ER status as risk factor for distance recurrence in patient T1N0M0 breast cancer. Clinical cancer research 2003 M0; 9(3): 223-309.

John GH, Langley P. Estimating continuous distributions in bayesian classifiers. In Proceedings of the Eleventh Conference on Unccertanity in Artificial Intelligence 1995; 338-345.

Keramatee K, Ghorbanian M, Abbasnia V, PazirehN, Alipour H, Effect of Flunixin as a Cox Inhibitor on Prevention and Cure of Breast Cancer in Female Wistar Rat, the Horizon of Medical Sciences 2010; 15 (4): 24-32.

Kim YS, Kanopler SN. Her-2 Overexpresion as a poor prognostic factor for patient with metastatic breast cancer undergoing high-dose chemotherapy with Autologus stemcell transplantation. Clinical cancer research. 2001 Dec; 7(12): 4003-12.

Kotsiantis SB. Supervised machin leaming: a reviw of classification techniques, informatica 31, 2007; 249-68.

Moller P, Wallin H, Knudesen LE. Oxidative stress associated psychological stress and life-style factor. Chem Bio Interact 1996; 102: 1-36.

Mousavi SM, Montazeri A, Mohagheghi MA, MousaviJarrahi A, Harirchi I, Najafi M, Ebrahimi M. Breast cancer in Iran: an epidemiological review. Breast J 2007; 13: 383-91.

Namiki M. Antioxidant /antimutagenes in foods. Crit Rev. food SciNutr 1990; 29: 273-300.

Nguyen AN, Lawley MJ, Hansen DP, Bowman RV, Clarke BE, Duhig EE, Colquist S. Symbolic rule-based classification of lung cancer stages from free-text pathology reports. J Am Med Inform Assoc 2010; 17(4):440-5.

Parkin DM, Bray F, Ferlay J, Pisani P. Global cancer statistics 2002. CA Cancer J Clin 2005; 55(2): 74-108.

Rosai J. Surgical pathology, Elsevier Inc. 9th edition Piladerphia 2004; 380-92.

Wang Rodrigez J, Cross K, Callagher S, Ojahanbin M, Armstrong JM. Male breast cancer correlation of ER, PR, Her-2 and P53 with treatment and survival a study of 65 cases. Modern pathology 2002 Aug; 15(8): 853-61. 7- Lipton A, Ali SM, Leitzel K. Eleuated serum Her-2 level predicts decrease response to hormone thrapy in metatatic breast cancer. Journal of clinical oncology 2002 Mar; 20(6): 1467- 72.

Wilson CM, Tobin S, Young RC. The exploding worldwide cancer burden: the impact of cancer on women. Int J Gynecol Cancer 2004; 14: 1-11.

Wilton CJ, Reeve JR, Going JJ, Cooke TG, Bortlett JM. Expression of the Her1-4 Family of receptor tyrosine kinase in breast cancer. Journal of pathology 2003; 200(3): 290-7.

Wuy Kan H, Chilar R. Prognostic value of plasma Her-2/Neu in African American and Hispanic woman with breast cancer. International journal of oncology 1999 Jun; 14(6): 1021-37. 13- Hehl EM. Opinion on the use of Anti-tumor druge trastuzumab (Herception) in patient with metastatic breast cancer. International journal of clinical pharmacology and thrapeutics. 2001 Nov; 39(4): 503-6.

Zhou Zh, Jiang Y. Medical diagnosis with C4.5 Rule preceded by artificial neural network ensemble. IEEE Trans InfTechnol Biomed 2003; 7(1): 37-42.

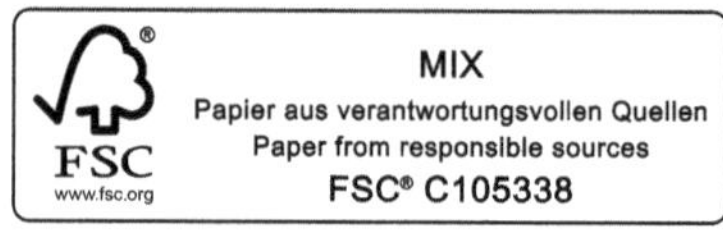

Printed by Books on Demand GmbH, Norderstedt / Germany